Fitness Calendar

Fill the days to keep track of your fitness goals

JANUARY

S	M	T	W	T	F	S
					1	2
3	4	5	6	7	8	9
10	11	12	13	14	15	16
17	18	19	20	21	22	23
24	25	26	27	28	29	30
31						

FEBRUARY

S	M	T	W	T	F	S
	1	2	3	4	5	6
7	8	9	10	11	12	13
14	15	16	17	18	19	20
21	22	23	24	25	26	27
28						

MARCH

S	M	T	W	T	F	S
	1	2	3	4	5	6
7	8	9	10	11	12	13
14	15	16	17	18	19	20
21	22	23	24	25	26	27
28	29	30	31			

APRIL

S	M	T	W	T	F	S
				1	2	3
4	5	6	7	8	9	10
11	12	13	14	15	16	17
18	19	20	21	22	23	24
25	26	27	28	29	30	

MAY

S	M	T	W	T	F	S
						1
2	3	4	5	6	7	8
9	10	11	12	13	14	15
16	17	18	19	20	21	22
23	24	25	26	27	28	29
30	31					

JUNE

S	M	T	W	T	F	S
		1	2	3	4	5
6	7	8	9	10	11	12
13	14	15	16	17	18	19
20	21	22	23	24	25	26
27	28	29	30			

JULY

S	M	T	W	T	F	S
				1	2	3
4	5	6	7	8	9	10
11	12	13	14	15	16	17
18	19	20	21	22	23	24
25	26	27	28	29	30	31

AUGUST

S	M	T	W	T	F	S
1	2	3	4	5	6	7
8	9	10	11	12	13	14
15	16	17	18	19	20	21
22	23	24	25	26	27	28
29	30	31				

SEPTEMBER

S	M	T	W	T	F	S
			1	2	3	4
5	6	7	8	9	10	11
12	13	14	15	16	17	18
19	20	21	22	23	24	25
26	27	28	29	30		

OCTOBER

S	M	T	W	T	F	S
					1	2
3	4	5	6	7	8	9
10	11	12	13	14	15	16
17	18	19	20	21	22	23
24	25	26	27	28	29	30
31						

NOVEMBER

S	M	T	W	T	F	S
	1	2	3	4	5	6
7	8	9	10	11	12	13
14	15	16	17	18	19	20
21	22	23	24	25	26	27
28	29	30				

DECEMBER

S	M	T	W	T	F	S
			1	2	3	4
5	6	7	8	9	10	11
12	13	14	15	16	17	18
19	20	21	22	23	24	25
26	27	28	29	30	31	

Monthly Planner

Month: _________ Year: _________

Monday	Tuesday	Wednesday	Thursday	Friday	Saturday	Sunday
☐	☐	☐	☐	☐	☐	☐
☐	☐	☐	☐	☐	☐	☐
☐	☐	☐	☐	☐	☐	☐
☐	☐	☐	☐	☐	☐	☐
☐	☐	☐	☐	☐	☐	☐

Notes:
____
____
____
____
____
____
____
____
____
____

BODY PROGRESS TRACKER

WAIST

Week 1: _______________

Week 2: _______________

Week 3: _______________

Week 4: _______________

ARMS

Week 1: _______________

Week 2: _______________

Week 3: _______________

Week 4: _______________

THIGHS

Week 1: _______________

Week 2: _______________

Week 3: _______________

Week 4: _______________

HIPS

Week 1: _______________

Week 2: _______________

Week 3: _______________

Week 4: _______________

Goal Tracker	Week 1:	Week 2:	Week 3:	Week 4:
DATE				
ARMS				
WAIST				
HIPS				
THIGHS				
WEIGHT				

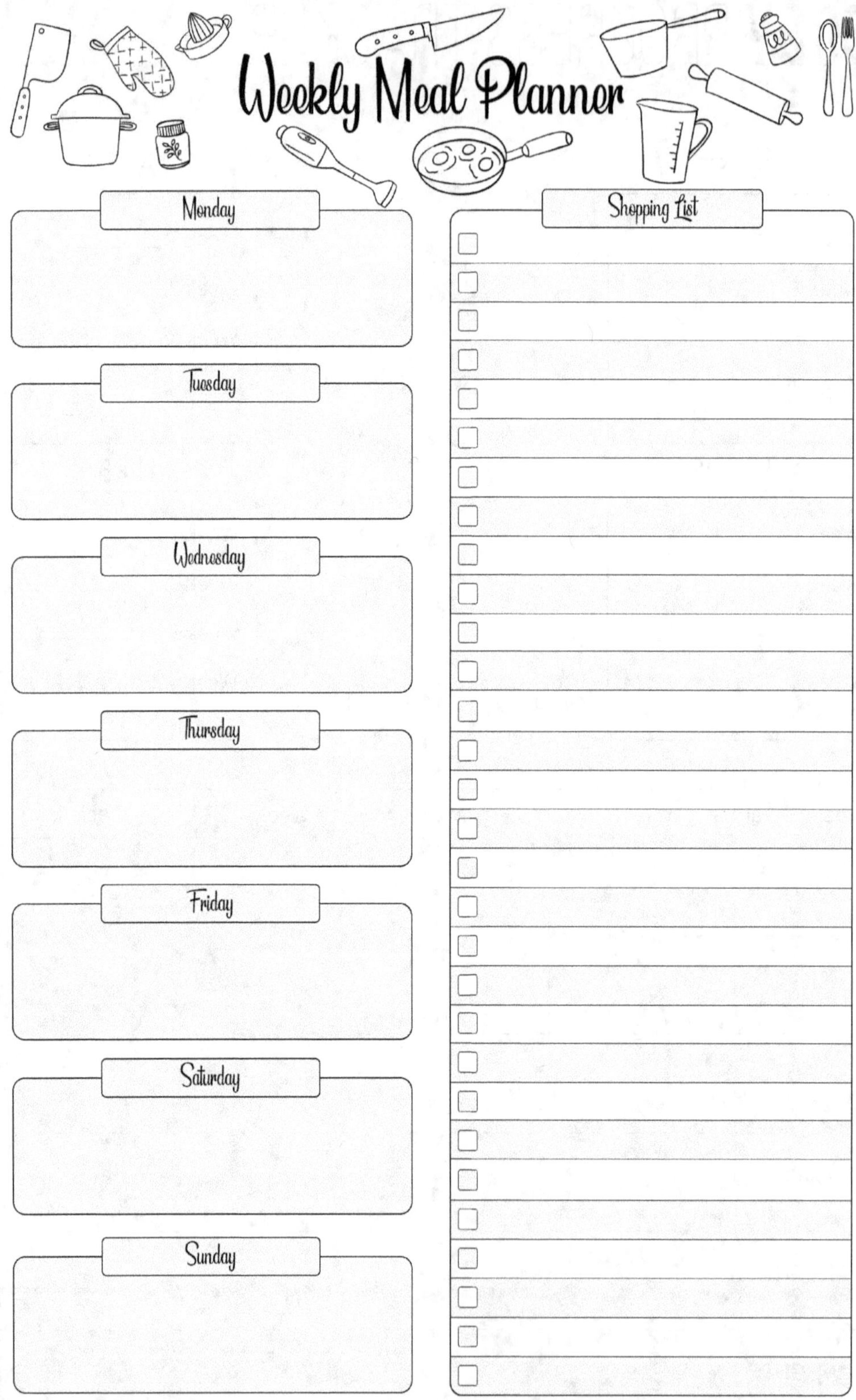

Weekly Meal Planner
Monday
Tuesday
Wednesday
Thursday
Friday
Saturday
Sunday
Shopping List

Weekly Meal Planner

Monday

Tuesday

Wednesday

Thursday

Friday

Saturday

Sunday

Shopping List

Weekly Meal Planner

Monday

Tuesday

Wednesday

Thursday

Friday

Saturday

Sunday

Shopping List

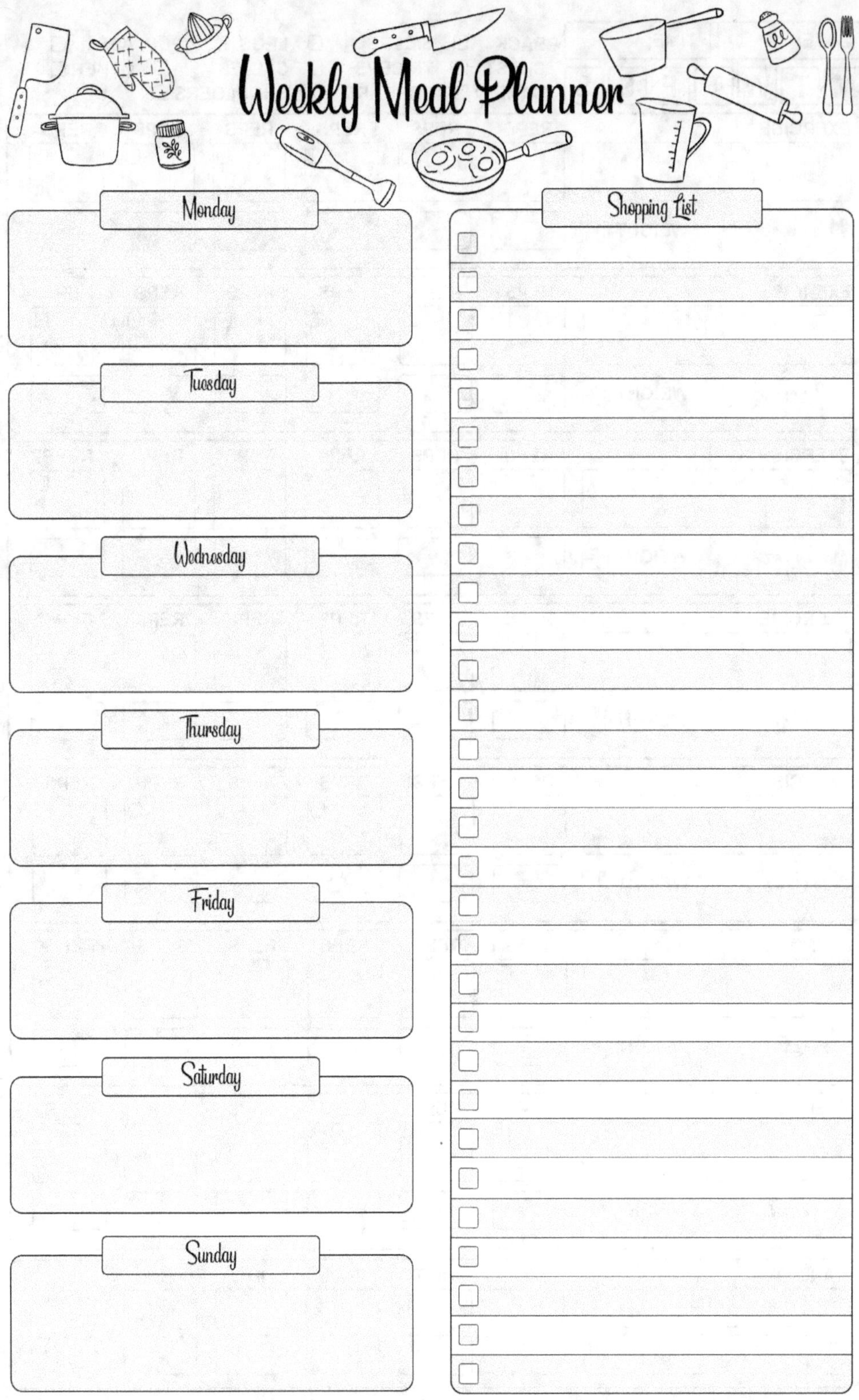

Weekly Meal Planner

Monday

Tuesday

Wednesday

Thursday

Friday

Saturday

Sunday

Shopping List

DATE: TIME:

M T W T F S S

BACK ☐ BICEPS ☐ LEGS ☐ ABS ☐
CHEST ☐ TRICEPS ☐ CALVES ☐ OTHER ☐
CARDIO ☐ FOREARMS ☐ SHOULDERS ☐

EXERCISE		REPS	REPS	REPS	REPS	REPS	REPS
1 234567	WEIGHT						

EXERCISE		REPS	REPS	REPS	REPS	REPS	REPS
1 **2** 34567	WEIGHT						

EXERCISE		REPS	REPS	REPS	REPS	REPS	REPS
12 **3** 4567	WEIGHT						

EXERCISE		REPS	REPS	REPS	REPS	REPS	REPS
123 **4** 567	WEIGHT						

EXERCISE		REPS	REPS	REPS	REPS	REPS	REPS
1234 **5** 67	WEIGHT						

EXERCISE		REPS	REPS	REPS	REPS	REPS	REPS
12345 **6** 7	WEIGHT						

EXERCISE		REPS	REPS	REPS	REPS	REPS	REPS
123456 **7**	WEIGHT						

CARDIO	TIME	DIST.	PACE	INT.	HR	
PRE-WORKOUT						
POST-WORKOUT						

DATE:

TIME:

M T W T F S S

BACK ☐ BICEPS ☐ LEGS ☐ ABS ☐
CHEST ☐ TRICEPS ☐ CALVES ☐ OTHER ☐
CARDIO ☐ FOREARMS ☐ SHOULDERS ☐

EXERCISE REPS REPS REPS REPS REPS REPS
1 2 3 4 5 6 7 WEIGHT

EXERCISE REPS REPS REPS REPS REPS REPS
1 **2** 3 4 5 6 7 WEIGHT

EXERCISE REPS REPS REPS REPS REPS REPS
1 2 **3** 4 5 6 7 WEIGHT

EXERCISE REPS REPS REPS REPS REPS REPS
1 2 3 **4** 5 6 7 WEIGHT

EXERCISE REPS REPS REPS REPS REPS REPS
1 2 3 4 **5** 6 7 WEIGHT

EXERCISE REPS REPS REPS REPS REPS REPS
1 2 3 4 5 **6** 7 WEIGHT

EXERCISE REPS REPS REPS REPS REPS REPS
1 2 3 4 5 6 **7** WEIGHT

CARDIO TIME DIST. PACE INT. HR
PRE-WORKOUT
POST-WORKOUT

EXERCISE	REPS	REPS	REPS	REPS	REPS	REPS
1 234567 WEIGHT						
1 **2** 34567 WEIGHT						
12 **3** 4567 WEIGHT						
123 **4** 567 WEIGHT						
1234 **5** 67 WEIGHT						
12345 **6** 7 WEIGHT						
123456 **7** WEIGHT						

CARDIO	TIME	DIST.	PACE	INT.	HR	
PRE-WORKOUT						
POST-WORKOUT						

DATE:

TIME:

M **T** **W** **T** **F** **S** **S**

BACK ☐ BICEPS ☐ LEGS ☐ ABS ☐
CHEST ☐ TRICEPS ☐ CALVES ☐ OTHER ☐
CARDIO ☐ FOREARMS ☐ SHOULDERS ☐

EXERCISE

REPS REPS REPS REPS REPS REPS

1 234567 WEIGHT

EXERCISE

REPS REPS REPS REPS REPS REPS

1 **2** 34567 WEIGHT

EXERCISE

REPS REPS REPS REPS REPS REPS

12 **3** 4567 WEIGHT

EXERCISE

REPS REPS REPS REPS REPS REPS

123 **4** 567 WEIGHT

EXERCISE

REPS REPS REPS REPS REPS REPS

1234 **5** 67 WEIGHT

EXERCISE

REPS REPS REPS REPS REPS REPS

12345 **6** 7 WEIGHT

EXERCISE

REPS REPS REPS REPS REPS REPS

123456 **7** WEIGHT

CARDIO TIME DIST. PACE INT. HR

PRE-WORKOUT

POST-WORKOUT

DATE: TIME:

M T W T F S S

BACK ☐ BICEPS ☐ LEGS ☐ ABS ☐
CHEST ☐ TRICEPS ☐ CALVES ☐ OTHER ☐
CARDIO ☐ FOREARMS ☐ SHOULDERS ☐

EXERCISE		REPS	REPS	REPS	REPS	REPS	REPS
1 2 3 4 5 6 7	WEIGHT						

EXERCISE		REPS	REPS	REPS	REPS	REPS	REPS
1 **2** 3 4 5 6 7	WEIGHT						

EXERCISE		REPS	REPS	REPS	REPS	REPS	REPS
1 2 **3** 4 5 6 7	WEIGHT						

EXERCISE		REPS	REPS	REPS	REPS	REPS	REPS
1 2 3 **4** 5 6 7	WEIGHT						

EXERCISE		REPS	REPS	REPS	REPS	REPS	REPS
1 2 3 4 **5** 6 7	WEIGHT						

EXERCISE		REPS	REPS	REPS	REPS	REPS	REPS
1 2 3 4 5 **6** 7	WEIGHT						

EXERCISE		REPS	REPS	REPS	REPS	REPS	REPS
1 2 3 4 5 6 **7**	WEIGHT						

CARDIO	TIME	DIST.	PACE	INT.	HR	
PRE-WORKOUT						
POST-WORKOUT						

DATE:	TIME:

M T W T F S S

BACK ☐	BICEPS ☐	LEGS ☐	ABS ☐
CHEST ☐	TRICEPS ☐	CALVES ☐	OTHER ☐
CARDIO ☐	FOREARMS ☐	SHOULDERS ☐	

EXERCISE

1 2 3 4 5 6 7   WEIGHT

REPS	REPS	REPS	REPS	REPS	REPS

EXERCISE

1 **2** 3 4 5 6 7   WEIGHT

REPS	REPS	REPS	REPS	REPS	REPS

EXERCISE

1 2 **3** 4 5 6 7   WEIGHT

REPS	REPS	REPS	REPS	REPS	REPS

EXERCISE

1 2 3 **4** 5 6 7   WEIGHT

REPS	REPS	REPS	REPS	REPS	REPS

EXERCISE

1 2 3 4 **5** 6 7   WEIGHT

REPS	REPS	REPS	REPS	REPS	REPS

EXERCISE

1 2 3 4 5 **6** 7   WEIGHT

REPS	REPS	REPS	REPS	REPS	REPS

EXERCISE

1 2 3 4 5 6 **7**   WEIGHT

REPS	REPS	REPS	REPS	REPS	REPS

CARDIO	TIME	DIST.	PACE	INT.	HR	
PRE-WORKOUT						
POST-WORKOUT						

DATE: | TIME:

M T W T F S S

BACK ☐ BICEPS ☐ LEGS ☐ ABS ☐
CHEST ☐ TRICEPS ☐ CALVES ☐ OTHER ☐
CARDIO ☐ FOREARMS ☐ SHOULDERS ☐

EXERCISE | REPS | REPS | REPS | REPS | REPS | REPS
1 234567 | WEIGHT

EXERCISE | REPS | REPS | REPS | REPS | REPS | REPS
1 **2** 34567 | WEIGHT

EXERCISE | REPS | REPS | REPS | REPS | REPS | REPS
12 **3** 4567 | WEIGHT

EXERCISE | REPS | REPS | REPS | REPS | REPS | REPS
123 **4** 567 | WEIGHT

EXERCISE | REPS | REPS | REPS | REPS | REPS | REPS
1234 **5** 67 | WEIGHT

EXERCISE | REPS | REPS | REPS | REPS | REPS | REPS
12345 **6** 7 | WEIGHT

EXERCISE | REPS | REPS | REPS | REPS | REPS | REPS
123456 **7** | WEIGHT

CARDIO | TIME | DIST. | PACE | INT. | HR
PRE-WORKOUT
POST-WORKOUT

Workout Log

DATE:	TIME:

M T W T F S S

- BACK ☐
- BICEPS ☐
- LEGS ☐
- ABS ☐
- CHEST ☐
- TRICEPS ☐
- CALVES ☐
- OTHER ☐
- CARDIO ☐
- FOREARMS ☐
- SHOULDERS ☐

EXERCISE 1 234567

WEIGHT	REPS	REPS	REPS	REPS	REPS	REPS

EXERCISE 1 2 34567

WEIGHT	REPS	REPS	REPS	REPS	REPS	REPS

EXERCISE 12 3 4567

WEIGHT	REPS	REPS	REPS	REPS	REPS	REPS

EXERCISE 123 4 567

WEIGHT	REPS	REPS	REPS	REPS	REPS	REPS

EXERCISE 1234 5 67

WEIGHT	REPS	REPS	REPS	REPS	REPS	REPS

EXERCISE 12345 6 7

WEIGHT	REPS	REPS	REPS	REPS	REPS	REPS

EXERCISE 123456 7

WEIGHT	REPS	REPS	REPS	REPS	REPS	REPS

CARDIO

	TIME	DIST.	PACE	INT.	HR
PRE-WORKOUT					
POST-WORKOUT					

<table>
<tr><td>DATE:</td><td>TIME:</td></tr>
</table>

M T W T F S S

BACK ☐ BICEPS ☐ LEGS ☐ ABS ☐
CHEST ☐ TRICEPS ☐ CALVES ☐ OTHER ☐
CARDIO ☐ FOREARMS ☐ SHOULDERS ☐

EXERCISE

1 2 3 4 5 6 7 WEIGHT

REPS	REPS	REPS	REPS	REPS	REPS

EXERCISE

1 **2** 3 4 5 6 7 WEIGHT

REPS	REPS	REPS	REPS	REPS	REPS

EXERCISE

1 2 **3** 4 5 6 7 WEIGHT

REPS	REPS	REPS	REPS	REPS	REPS

EXERCISE

1 2 3 **4** 5 6 7 WEIGHT

REPS	REPS	REPS	REPS	REPS	REPS

EXERCISE

1 2 3 4 **5** 6 7 WEIGHT

REPS	REPS	REPS	REPS	REPS	REPS

EXERCISE

1 2 3 4 5 **6** 7 WEIGHT

REPS	REPS	REPS	REPS	REPS	REPS

EXERCISE

1 2 3 4 5 6 **7** WEIGHT

REPS	REPS	REPS	REPS	REPS	REPS

CARDIO

	TIME	DIST.	PACE	INT.	HR
PRE-WORKOUT					
POST-WORKOUT					

DATE: TIME:

M T W T F S S

BACK ☐   BICEPS ☐   LEGS ☐   ABS ☐
CHEST ☐   TRICEPS ☐   CALVES ☐   OTHER ☐
CARDIO ☐   FOREARMS ☐   SHOULDERS ☐

EXERCISE — REPS REPS REPS REPS REPS REPS

1 2 3 4 5 6 7   WEIGHT

EXERCISE — REPS REPS REPS REPS REPS REPS

1 **2** 3 4 5 6 7   WEIGHT

EXERCISE — REPS REPS REPS REPS REPS REPS

1 2 **3** 4 5 6 7   WEIGHT

EXERCISE — REPS REPS REPS REPS REPS REPS

1 2 3 **4** 5 6 7   WEIGHT

EXERCISE — REPS REPS REPS REPS REPS REPS

1 2 3 4 **5** 6 7   WEIGHT

EXERCISE — REPS REPS REPS REPS REPS REPS

1 2 3 4 5 **6** 7   WEIGHT

EXERCISE — REPS REPS REPS REPS REPS REPS

1 2 3 4 5 6 **7**   WEIGHT

CARDIO   TIME   DIST.   PACE   INT.   HR

PRE-WORKOUT

POST-WORKOUT

| DATE: | TIME: |

M T W T F S S

BACK ☐ BICEPS ☐ LEGS ☐ ABS ☐
CHEST ☐ TRICEPS ☐ CALVES ☐ OTHER ☐
CARDIO ☐ FOREARMS ☐ SHOULDERS ☐

EXERCISE | REPS | REPS | REPS | REPS | REPS | REPS

1 234567 WEIGHT

EXERCISE | REPS | REPS | REPS | REPS | REPS | REPS

1 **2** 34567 WEIGHT

EXERCISE | REPS | REPS | REPS | REPS | REPS | REPS

12 **3** 4567 WEIGHT

EXERCISE | REPS | REPS | REPS | REPS | REPS | REPS

123 **4** 567 WEIGHT

EXERCISE | REPS | REPS | REPS | REPS | REPS | REPS

1234 **5** 67 WEIGHT

EXERCISE | REPS | REPS | REPS | REPS | REPS | REPS

12345 **6** 7 WEIGHT

EXERCISE | REPS | REPS | REPS | REPS | REPS | REPS

123456 **7** WEIGHT

CARDIO | TIME | DIST. | PACE | INT. | HR

PRE-WORKOUT

POST-WORKOUT

DATE:
TIME:
M T W T F S S

BACK ☐ BICEPS ☐ LEGS ☐ ABS ☐
CHEST ☐ TRICEPS ☐ CALVES ☐ OTHER ☐
CARDIO ☐ FOREARMS ☐ SHOULDERS ☐

EXERCISE
REPS REPS REPS REPS REPS REPS
1 234567 WEIGHT

EXERCISE
REPS REPS REPS REPS REPS REPS
1 2 34567 WEIGHT

EXERCISE
REPS REPS REPS REPS REPS REPS
12 3 4567 WEIGHT

EXERCISE
REPS REPS REPS REPS REPS REPS
123 4 567 WEIGHT

EXERCISE
REPS REPS REPS REPS REPS REPS
1234 5 67 WEIGHT

EXERCISE
REPS REPS REPS REPS REPS REPS
12345 6 7 WEIGHT

EXERCISE
REPS REPS REPS REPS REPS REPS
123456 7 WEIGHT

CARDIO
TIME DIST. PACE INT. HR
PRE-WORKOUT
POST-WORKOUT

| DATE: | TIME: |

M T W T F S S

- BACK ☐ BICEPS ☐ LEGS ☐ ABS ☐
- CHEST ☐ TRICEPS ☐ CALVES ☐ OTHER ☐
- CARDIO ☐ FOREARMS ☐ SHOULDERS ☐

EXERCISE

REPS	REPS	REPS	REPS	REPS	REPS

1 2 3 4 5 6 7 WEIGHT

EXERCISE

REPS	REPS	REPS	REPS	REPS	REPS

1 **2** 3 4 5 6 7 WEIGHT

EXERCISE

REPS	REPS	REPS	REPS	REPS	REPS

1 2 **3** 4 5 6 7 WEIGHT

EXERCISE

REPS	REPS	REPS	REPS	REPS	REPS

1 2 3 **4** 5 6 7 WEIGHT

EXERCISE

REPS	REPS	REPS	REPS	REPS	REPS

1 2 3 4 **5** 6 7 WEIGHT

EXERCISE

REPS	REPS	REPS	REPS	REPS	REPS

1 2 3 4 5 **6** 7 WEIGHT

EXERCISE

REPS	REPS	REPS	REPS	REPS	REPS

1 2 3 4 5 6 **7** WEIGHT

CARDIO

	TIME	DIST.	PACE	INT.	HR
PRE-WORKOUT					
POST-WORKOUT					

DATE:	TIME:	BACK ☐	BICEPS ☐	LEGS ☐	ABS ☐
		CHEST ☐	TRICEPS ☐	CALVES ☐	OTHER ☐
M T W T F S S		CARDIO ☐	FOREARMS ☐	SHOULDERS ☐	

EXERCISE

1 2 3 4 5 6 7 — WEIGHT | REPS | REPS | REPS | REPS | REPS | REPS

EXERCISE

1 **2** 3 4 5 6 7 — WEIGHT | REPS | REPS | REPS | REPS | REPS | REPS

EXERCISE

1 2 **3** 4 5 6 7 — WEIGHT | REPS | REPS | REPS | REPS | REPS | REPS

EXERCISE

1 2 3 **4** 5 6 7 — WEIGHT | REPS | REPS | REPS | REPS | REPS | REPS

EXERCISE

1 2 3 4 **5** 6 7 — WEIGHT | REPS | REPS | REPS | REPS | REPS | REPS

EXERCISE

1 2 3 4 5 **6** 7 — WEIGHT | REPS | REPS | REPS | REPS | REPS | REPS

EXERCISE

1 2 3 4 5 6 **7** — WEIGHT | REPS | REPS | REPS | REPS | REPS | REPS

CARDIO	TIME	DIST.	PACE	INT.	HR	
PRE-WORKOUT						
POST-WORKOUT						

<table>
<tr><td>DATE:</td><td>TIME:</td><td colspan="2">BACK ☐   BICEPS ☐   LEGS ☐   ABS ☐</td></tr>
<tr><td colspan="2">M T W T F S S</td><td colspan="2">CHEST ☐   TRICEPS ☐   CALVES ☐   OTHER ☐
CARDIO ☐   FOREARMS ☐   SHOULDERS ☐</td></tr>
</table>

EXERCISE

1 234567   WEIGHT

REPS	REPS	REPS	REPS	REPS	REPS

EXERCISE

1 **2** 34567   WEIGHT

REPS	REPS	REPS	REPS	REPS	REPS

EXERCISE

12 **3** 4567   WEIGHT

REPS	REPS	REPS	REPS	REPS	REPS

EXERCISE

123 **4** 567   WEIGHT

REPS	REPS	REPS	REPS	REPS	REPS

EXERCISE

1234 **5** 67   WEIGHT

REPS	REPS	REPS	REPS	REPS	REPS

EXERCISE

12345 **6** 7   WEIGHT

REPS	REPS	REPS	REPS	REPS	REPS

EXERCISE

123456 **7**   WEIGHT

REPS	REPS	REPS	REPS	REPS	REPS

CARDIO

	TIME	DIST.	PACE	INT.	HR
PRE-WORKOUT					
POST-WORKOUT					

DATE: TIME:

M T W T F S S

BACK ☐   BICEPS ☐   LEGS ☐   ABS ☐
CHEST ☐   TRICEPS ☐   CALVES ☐   OTHER ☐
CARDIO ☐   FOREARMS ☐   SHOULDERS ☐

EXERCISE

1 2 3 4 5 6 7   WEIGHT

REPS ☐	REPS ☐	REPS ☐	REPS ☐	REPS ☐	REPS ☐

EXERCISE

1 **2** 3 4 5 6 7   WEIGHT

REPS ☐	REPS ☐	REPS ☐	REPS ☐	REPS ☐	REPS ☐

EXERCISE

1 2 **3** 4 5 6 7   WEIGHT

REPS ☐	REPS ☐	REPS ☐	REPS ☐	REPS ☐	REPS ☐

EXERCISE

1 2 3 **4** 5 6 7   WEIGHT

REPS ☐	REPS ☐	REPS ☐	REPS ☐	REPS ☐	REPS ☐

EXERCISE

1 2 3 4 **5** 6 7   WEIGHT

REPS ☐	REPS ☐	REPS ☐	REPS ☐	REPS ☐	REPS ☐

EXERCISE

1 2 3 4 5 **6** 7   WEIGHT

REPS ☐	REPS ☐	REPS ☐	REPS ☐	REPS ☐	REPS ☐

EXERCISE

1 2 3 4 5 6 **7**   WEIGHT

REPS ☐	REPS ☐	REPS ☐	REPS ☐	REPS ☐	REPS ☐

CARDIO	TIME	DIST.	PACE	INT.	HR	
PRE-WORKOUT						☺ 😀
POST-WORKOUT						☹ ☺

<table>
<tr><td>DATE:</td><td>TIME:</td><td colspan="2">BACK ☐   BICEPS ☐   LEGS ☐   ABS ☐</td></tr>
<tr><td colspan="2">M T W T F S S</td><td colspan="2">CHEST ☐   TRICEPS ☐   CALVES ☐   OTHER ☐
CARDIO ☐   FOREARMS ☐   SHOULDERS ☐</td></tr>
</table>

EXERCISE	REPS ☐	REPS ☐	REPS ☐	REPS ☐	REPS ☐	REPS ☐
1 2 3 4 5 6 7 WEIGHT					

EXERCISE	REPS ☐	REPS ☐	REPS ☐	REPS ☐	REPS ☐	REPS ☐
1 **2** 3 4 5 6 7 WEIGHT					

EXERCISE	REPS ☐	REPS ☐	REPS ☐	REPS ☐	REPS ☐	REPS ☐
1 2 **3** 4 5 6 7 WEIGHT					

EXERCISE	REPS ☐	REPS ☐	REPS ☐	REPS ☐	REPS ☐	REPS ☐
1 2 3 **4** 5 6 7 WEIGHT					

EXERCISE	REPS ☐	REPS ☐	REPS ☐	REPS ☐	REPS ☐	REPS ☐
1 2 3 4 **5** 6 7 WEIGHT					

EXERCISE	REPS ☐	REPS ☐	REPS ☐	REPS ☐	REPS ☐	REPS ☐
1 2 3 4 5 **6** 7 WEIGHT					

EXERCISE	REPS ☐	REPS ☐	REPS ☐	REPS ☐	REPS ☐	REPS ☐
1 2 3 4 5 6 **7** WEIGHT					

CARDIO	TIME	DIST.	PACE	INT.	HR
PRE-WORKOUT				
POST-WORKOUT				

DATE: TIME:

M **T** **W** **T** **F** **S** **S**

BACK ☐   BICEPS ☐   LEGS ☐   ABS ☐
CHEST ☐   TRICEPS ☐   CALVES ☐   OTHER ☐
CARDIO ☐   FOREARMS ☐   SHOULDERS ☐

EXERCISE

1 2 3 4 5 6 7   WEIGHT

REPS | REPS | REPS | REPS | REPS | REPS

EXERCISE

1 **2** 3 4 5 6 7   WEIGHT

REPS | REPS | REPS | REPS | REPS | REPS

EXERCISE

1 2 **3** 4 5 6 7   WEIGHT

REPS | REPS | REPS | REPS | REPS | REPS

EXERCISE

1 2 3 **4** 5 6 7   WEIGHT

REPS | REPS | REPS | REPS | REPS | REPS

EXERCISE

1 2 3 4 **5** 6 7   WEIGHT

REPS | REPS | REPS | REPS | REPS | REPS

EXERCISE

1 2 3 4 5 **6** 7   WEIGHT

REPS | REPS | REPS | REPS | REPS | REPS

EXERCISE

1 2 3 4 5 6 **7**   WEIGHT

REPS | REPS | REPS | REPS | REPS | REPS

CARDIO

CARDIO	TIME	DIST.	PACE	INT.	HR
PRE-WORKOUT					
POST-WORKOUT					

DATE:
TIME:
M T W T F S S
BACK ☐   BICEPS ☐   LEGS ☐   ABS ☐
CHEST ☐   TRICEPS ☐   CALVES ☐   OTHER ☐
CARDIO ☐   FOREARMS ☐   SHOULDERS ☐

EXERCISE
1 234567   WEIGHT   REPS REPS REPS REPS REPS REPS

EXERCISE
1 2 34567   WEIGHT   REPS REPS REPS REPS REPS REPS

EXERCISE
12 3 4567   WEIGHT   REPS REPS REPS REPS REPS REPS

EXERCISE
123 4 567   WEIGHT   REPS REPS REPS REPS REPS REPS

EXERCISE
1234 5 67   WEIGHT   REPS REPS REPS REPS REPS REPS

EXERCISE
12345 6 7   WEIGHT   REPS REPS REPS REPS REPS REPS

EXERCISE
123456 7   WEIGHT   REPS REPS REPS REPS REPS REPS

CARDIO   TIME DIST. PACE INT. HR
PRE-WORKOUT
POST-WORKOUT

DATE: | TIME:

M **T** **W** **T** **F** **S** **S**

BACK ☐ BICEPS ☐ LEGS ☐ ABS ☐
CHEST ☐ TRICEPS ☐ CALVES ☐ OTHER ☐
CARDIO ☐ FOREARMS ☐ SHOULDERS ☐

EXERCISE
REPS REPS REPS REPS REPS REPS
1 2 3 4 5 6 7 WEIGHT

EXERCISE
REPS REPS REPS REPS REPS REPS
1 **2** 3 4 5 6 7 WEIGHT

EXERCISE
REPS REPS REPS REPS REPS REPS
1 2 **3** 4 5 6 7 WEIGHT

EXERCISE
REPS REPS REPS REPS REPS REPS
1 2 3 **4** 5 6 7 WEIGHT

EXERCISE
REPS REPS REPS REPS REPS REPS
1 2 3 4 **5** 6 7 WEIGHT

EXERCISE
REPS REPS REPS REPS REPS REPS
1 2 3 4 5 **6** 7 WEIGHT

EXERCISE
REPS REPS REPS REPS REPS REPS
1 2 3 4 5 6 **7** WEIGHT

CARDIO
TIME DIST. PACE INT. HR
PRE-WORKOUT
POST-WORKOUT

DATE: | TIME:

M T W T F S S

BACK ☐   BICEPS ☐   LEGS ☐   ABS ☐
CHEST ☐   TRICEPS ☐   CALVES ☐   OTHER ☐
CARDIO ☐   FOREARMS ☐   SHOULDERS ☐

EXERCISE   REPS REPS REPS REPS REPS REPS

1 234567   WEIGHT

EXERCISE   REPS REPS REPS REPS REPS REPS

1 **2** 34567   WEIGHT

EXERCISE   REPS REPS REPS REPS REPS REPS

12 **3** 4567   WEIGHT

EXERCISE   REPS REPS REPS REPS REPS REPS

123 **4** 567   WEIGHT

EXERCISE   REPS REPS REPS REPS REPS REPS

1234 **5** 67   WEIGHT

EXERCISE   REPS REPS REPS REPS REPS REPS

12345 **6** 7   WEIGHT

EXERCISE   REPS REPS REPS REPS REPS REPS

123456 **7**   WEIGHT

CARDIO   TIME   DIST.   PACE   INT.   HR

PRE-WORKOUT

POST-WORKOUT

DATE:
TIME:
M T W T F S S
BACK ☐ BICEPS ☐ LEGS ☐ ABS ☐
CHEST ☐ TRICEPS ☐ CALVES ☐ OTHER ☐
CARDIO ☐ FOREARMS ☐ SHOULDERS ☐

EXERCISE
REPS REPS REPS REPS REPS REPS
1 234567 WEIGHT

EXERCISE
REPS REPS REPS REPS REPS REPS
1 2 34567 WEIGHT

EXERCISE
REPS REPS REPS REPS REPS REPS
12 3 4567 WEIGHT

EXERCISE
REPS REPS REPS REPS REPS REPS
123 4 567 WEIGHT

EXERCISE
REPS REPS REPS REPS REPS REPS
1234 5 67 WEIGHT

EXERCISE
REPS REPS REPS REPS REPS REPS
12345 6 7 WEIGHT

EXERCISE
REPS REPS REPS REPS REPS REPS
123456 7 WEIGHT

CARDIO TIME DIST. PACE INT. HR
PRE-WORKOUT
POST-WORKOUT

DATE: ___ TIME: ___

M T W T F S S

BACK ☐ BICEPS ☐ LEGS ☐ ABS ☐
CHEST ☐ TRICEPS ☐ CALVES ☐ OTHER ☐
CARDIO ☐ FOREARMS ☐ SHOULDERS ☐

EXERCISE	REPS	REPS	REPS	REPS	REPS	REPS
1 234567 WEIGHT						

EXERCISE	REPS	REPS	REPS	REPS	REPS	REPS
1 **2** 34567 WEIGHT						

EXERCISE	REPS	REPS	REPS	REPS	REPS	REPS
12 **3** 4567 WEIGHT						

EXERCISE	REPS	REPS	REPS	REPS	REPS	REPS
123 **4** 567 WEIGHT						

EXERCISE	REPS	REPS	REPS	REPS	REPS	REPS
1234 **5** 67 WEIGHT						

EXERCISE	REPS	REPS	REPS	REPS	REPS	REPS
12345 **6** 7 WEIGHT						

EXERCISE	REPS	REPS	REPS	REPS	REPS	REPS
123456 **7** WEIGHT						

CARDIO	TIME	DIST.	PACE	INT.	HR
PRE-WORKOUT					
POST-WORKOUT					

DATE: TIME:

M **T** **W** **T** **F** **S** **S**

BACK ☐   BICEPS ☐   LEGS ☐   ABS ☐
CHEST ☐   TRICEPS ☐   CALVES ☐   OTHER ☐
CARDIO ☐   FOREARMS ☐   SHOULDERS ☐

EXERCISE	REPS	REPS	REPS	REPS	REPS	REPS
1 2 3 4 5 6 7 WEIGHT						

EXERCISE	REPS	REPS	REPS	REPS	REPS	REPS
1 **2** 3 4 5 6 7 WEIGHT						

EXERCISE	REPS	REPS	REPS	REPS	REPS	REPS
1 2 **3** 4 5 6 7 WEIGHT						

EXERCISE	REPS	REPS	REPS	REPS	REPS	REPS
1 2 3 **4** 5 6 7 WEIGHT						

EXERCISE	REPS	REPS	REPS	REPS	REPS	REPS
1 2 3 4 **5** 6 7 WEIGHT						

EXERCISE	REPS	REPS	REPS	REPS	REPS	REPS
1 2 3 4 5 **6** 7 WEIGHT						

EXERCISE	REPS	REPS	REPS	REPS	REPS	REPS
1 2 3 4 5 6 **7** WEIGHT						

CARDIO	TIME	DIST.	PACE	INT.	HR	
PRE-WORKOUT						
POST-WORKOUT						

DATE:	TIME:	BACK ☐	BICEPS ☐	LEGS ☐	ABS ☐
CHEST ☐	TRICEPS ☐	CALVES ☐	OTHER ☐
CARDIO ☐	FOREARMS ☐	SHOULDERS ☐

M T W T F S S

EXERCISE

1 2 3 4 5 6 7 — WEIGHT

| REPS | REPS | REPS | REPS | REPS | REPS |

EXERCISE

1 **2** 3 4 5 6 7 — WEIGHT

| REPS | REPS | REPS | REPS | REPS | REPS |

EXERCISE

1 2 **3** 4 5 6 7 — WEIGHT

| REPS | REPS | REPS | REPS | REPS | REPS |

EXERCISE

1 2 3 **4** 5 6 7 — WEIGHT

| REPS | REPS | REPS | REPS | REPS | REPS |

EXERCISE

1 2 3 4 **5** 6 7 — WEIGHT

| REPS | REPS | REPS | REPS | REPS | REPS |

EXERCISE

1 2 3 4 5 **6** 7 — WEIGHT

| REPS | REPS | REPS | REPS | REPS | REPS |

EXERCISE

1 2 3 4 5 6 **7** — WEIGHT

| REPS | REPS | REPS | REPS | REPS | REPS |

CARDIO

	TIME	DIST.	PACE	INT.	HR
PRE-WORKOUT					
POST-WORKOUT					

DATE:	TIME:

M T W T F S S

BACK ☐	BICEPS ☐	LEGS ☐	ABS ☐
CHEST ☐	TRICEPS ☐	CALVES ☐	OTHER ☐
CARDIO ☐	FOREARMS ☐	SHOULDERS ☐	

EXERCISE

1 234567   WEIGHT

REPS ☐	REPS ☐	REPS ☐	REPS ☐	REPS ☐	REPS ☐

EXERCISE

1 **2** 34567   WEIGHT

REPS ☐	REPS ☐	REPS ☐	REPS ☐	REPS ☐	REPS ☐

EXERCISE

12 **3** 4567   WEIGHT

REPS ☐	REPS ☐	REPS ☐	REPS ☐	REPS ☐	REPS ☐

EXERCISE

123 **4** 567   WEIGHT

REPS ☐	REPS ☐	REPS ☐	REPS ☐	REPS ☐	REPS ☐

EXERCISE

1234 **5** 67   WEIGHT

REPS ☐	REPS ☐	REPS ☐	REPS ☐	REPS ☐	REPS ☐

EXERCISE

12345 **6** 7   WEIGHT

REPS ☐	REPS ☐	REPS ☐	REPS ☐	REPS ☐	REPS ☐

EXERCISE

123456 **7**   WEIGHT

REPS ☐	REPS ☐	REPS ☐	REPS ☐	REPS ☐	REPS ☐

CARDIO	TIME	DIST.	PACE	INT.	HR	
PRE-WORKOUT						
POST-WORKOUT						

DATE:
TIME:
M T W T F S S
BACK ☐   BICEPS ☐   LEGS ☐   ABS ☐
CHEST ☐   TRICEPS ☐   CALVES ☐   OTHER ☐
CARDIO ☐   FOREARMS ☐   SHOULDERS ☐

EXERCISE
REPS REPS REPS REPS REPS REPS
1 234567   WEIGHT

EXERCISE
REPS REPS REPS REPS REPS REPS
1 2 34567   WEIGHT

EXERCISE
REPS REPS REPS REPS REPS REPS
12 3 4567   WEIGHT

EXERCISE
REPS REPS REPS REPS REPS REPS
123 4 567   WEIGHT

EXERCISE
REPS REPS REPS REPS REPS REPS
1234 5 67   WEIGHT

EXERCISE
REPS REPS REPS REPS REPS REPS
12345 6 7   WEIGHT

EXERCISE
REPS REPS REPS REPS REPS REPS
123456 7   WEIGHT

CARDIO   TIME   DIST.   PACE   INT.   HR
PRE-WORKOUT
POST-WORKOUT

Monthly Planner

Month: _______ Year: _______

Monday	Tuesday	Wednesday	Thursday	Friday	Saturday	Sunday
☐	☐	☐	☐	☐	☐	☐
☐	☐	☐	☐	☐	☐	☐
☐	☐	☐	☐	☐	☐	☐
☐	☐	☐	☐	☐	☐	☐
☐	☐	☐	☐	☐	☐	☐

Notes:

BODY PROGRESS TRACKER

WAIST

Week 1: _______________

Week 2: _______________

Week 3: _______________

Week 4: _______________

ARMS

Week 1: _______________

Week 2: _______________

Week 3: _______________

Week 4: _______________

THIGHS

Week 1: _______________

Week 2: _______________

Week 3: _______________

Week 4: _______________

HIPS

Week 1: _______________

Week 2: _______________

Week 3: _______________

Week 4: _______________

Goal Tracker	Week 1:	Week 2:	Week 3:	Week 4:
DATE				
ARMS				
WAIST				
HIPS				
THIGHS				
WEIGHT				

Weekly Meal Planner

Monday

Tuesday

Wednesday

Thursday

Friday

Saturday

Sunday

Shopping List

Weekly Meal Planner

Monday

Tuesday

Wednesday

Thursday

Friday

Saturday

Sunday

Shopping List

Weekly Meal Planner

Monday

Tuesday

Wednesday

Thursday

Friday

Saturday

Sunday

Shopping List

Weekly Meal Planner

Monday

Tuesday

Wednesday

Thursday

Friday

Saturday

Sunday

Shopping List

DATE: TIME:

M **T** **W** **T** **F** **S** **S**

BACK ☐   BICEPS ☐   LEGS ☐   ABS ☐
CHEST ☐   TRICEPS ☐   CALVES ☐   OTHER ☐
CARDIO ☐   FOREARMS ☐   SHOULDERS ☐

EXERCISE	REPS	REPS	REPS	REPS	REPS	REPS
1 234567 WEIGHT						
1 **2** 34567 WEIGHT						
12 **3** 4567 WEIGHT						
123 **4** 567 WEIGHT						
1234 **5** 67 WEIGHT						
12345 **6** 7 WEIGHT						
123456 **7** WEIGHT						

CARDIO	TIME	DIST.	PACE	INT.	HR	
PRE-WORKOUT						
POST-WORKOUT						

DATE: TIME:

| M | T | W | T | F | S | S |

BACK ☐ BICEPS ☐ LEGS ☐ ABS ☐
CHEST ☐ TRICEPS ☐ CALVES ☐ OTHER ☐
CARDIO ☐ FOREARMS ☐ SHOULDERS ☐

EXERCISE

REPS ☐ REPS ☐ REPS ☐ REPS ☐ REPS ☐ REPS ☐

1 2 3 4 5 6 7 WEIGHT

EXERCISE

REPS ☐ REPS ☐ REPS ☐ REPS ☐ REPS ☐ REPS ☐

1 **2** 3 4 5 6 7 WEIGHT

EXERCISE

REPS ☐ REPS ☐ REPS ☐ REPS ☐ REPS ☐ REPS ☐

1 2 **3** 4 5 6 7 WEIGHT

EXERCISE

REPS ☐ REPS ☐ REPS ☐ REPS ☐ REPS ☐ REPS ☐

1 2 3 **4** 5 6 7 WEIGHT

EXERCISE

REPS ☐ REPS ☐ REPS ☐ REPS ☐ REPS ☐ REPS ☐

1 2 3 4 **5** 6 7 WEIGHT

EXERCISE

REPS ☐ REPS ☐ REPS ☐ REPS ☐ REPS ☐ REPS ☐

1 2 3 4 5 **6** 7 WEIGHT

EXERCISE

REPS ☐ REPS ☐ REPS ☐ REPS ☐ REPS ☐ REPS ☐

1 2 3 4 5 6 **7** WEIGHT

CARDIO TIME DIST. PACE INT. HR

PRE-WORKOUT

POST-WORKOUT

DATE: TIME:

BACK ☐   BICEPS ☐   LEGS ☐   ABS ☐
CHEST ☐   TRICEPS ☐   CALVES ☐   OTHER ☐
CARDIO ☐   FOREARMS ☐   SHOULDERS ☐

M T W T F S S

EXERCISE
1 234567   WEIGHT   REPS | REPS | REPS | REPS | REPS | REPS

EXERCISE
1 **2** 34567   WEIGHT   REPS | REPS | REPS | REPS | REPS | REPS

EXERCISE
12 **3** 4567   WEIGHT   REPS | REPS | REPS | REPS | REPS | REPS

EXERCISE
123 **4** 567   WEIGHT   REPS | REPS | REPS | REPS | REPS | REPS

EXERCISE
1234 **5** 67   WEIGHT   REPS | REPS | REPS | REPS | REPS | REPS

EXERCISE
12345 **6** 7   WEIGHT   REPS | REPS | REPS | REPS | REPS | REPS

EXERCISE
123456 **7**   WEIGHT   REPS | REPS | REPS | REPS | REPS | REPS

CARDIO
	TIME	DIST.	PACE	INT.	HR
PRE-WORKOUT					
POST-WORKOUT					

DATE: | TIME:

M **T** **W** **T** **F** **S** **S**

BACK ☐   BICEPS ☐   LEGS ☐   ABS ☐
CHEST ☐   TRICEPS ☐   CALVES ☐   OTHER ☐
CARDIO ☐   FOREARMS ☐   SHOULDERS ☐

EXERCISE

1 234567   WEIGHT

REPS	REPS	REPS	REPS	REPS	REPS

EXERCISE

1 **2** 34567   WEIGHT

REPS	REPS	REPS	REPS	REPS	REPS

EXERCISE

12 **3** 4567   WEIGHT

REPS	REPS	REPS	REPS	REPS	REPS

EXERCISE

123 **4** 567   WEIGHT

REPS	REPS	REPS	REPS	REPS	REPS

EXERCISE

1234 **5** 67   WEIGHT

REPS	REPS	REPS	REPS	REPS	REPS

EXERCISE

12345 **6** 7   WEIGHT

REPS	REPS	REPS	REPS	REPS	REPS

EXERCISE

123456 **7**   WEIGHT

REPS	REPS	REPS	REPS	REPS	REPS

CARDIO

	TIME	DIST.	PACE	INT.	HR
PRE-WORKOUT					
POST-WORKOUT					

DATE: TIME:

M T W T F S S

BACK ☐   BICEPS ☐   LEGS ☐   ABS ☐
CHEST ☐   TRICEPS ☐   CALVES ☐   OTHER ☐
CARDIO ☐   FOREARMS ☐   SHOULDERS ☐

EXERCISE	REPS	REPS	REPS	REPS	REPS	REPS
1 234567 WEIGHT						

EXERCISE	REPS	REPS	REPS	REPS	REPS	REPS
1 **2** 34567 WEIGHT						

EXERCISE	REPS	REPS	REPS	REPS	REPS	REPS
12 **3** 4567 WEIGHT						

EXERCISE	REPS	REPS	REPS	REPS	REPS	REPS
123 **4** 567 WEIGHT						

EXERCISE	REPS	REPS	REPS	REPS	REPS	REPS
1234 **5** 67 WEIGHT						

EXERCISE	REPS	REPS	REPS	REPS	REPS	REPS
12345 **6** 7 WEIGHT						

EXERCISE	REPS	REPS	REPS	REPS	REPS	REPS
123456 **7** WEIGHT						

CARDIO	TIME	DIST.	PACE	INT.	HR	
PRE-WORKOUT						
POST-WORKOUT						

DATE: | TIME:

M **T** **W** **T** **F** **S** **S**

BACK ☐ BICEPS ☐ LEGS ☐ ABS ☐
CHEST ☐ TRICEPS ☐ CALVES ☐ OTHER ☐
CARDIO ☐ FOREARMS ☐ SHOULDERS ☐

EXERCISE	REPS	REPS	REPS	REPS	REPS	REPS
1 2 3 4 5 6 7 WEIGHT						

EXERCISE	REPS	REPS	REPS	REPS	REPS	REPS
1 **2** 3 4 5 6 7 WEIGHT						

EXERCISE	REPS	REPS	REPS	REPS	REPS	REPS
1 2 **3** 4 5 6 7 WEIGHT						

EXERCISE	REPS	REPS	REPS	REPS	REPS	REPS
1 2 3 **4** 5 6 7 WEIGHT						

EXERCISE	REPS	REPS	REPS	REPS	REPS	REPS
1 2 3 4 **5** 6 7 WEIGHT						

EXERCISE	REPS	REPS	REPS	REPS	REPS	REPS
1 2 3 4 5 **6** 7 WEIGHT						

EXERCISE	REPS	REPS	REPS	REPS	REPS	REPS
1 2 3 4 5 6 **7** WEIGHT						

CARDIO	TIME	DIST.	PACE	INT.	HR	
PRE-WORKOUT						
POST-WORKOUT						

| DATE: | TIME: |

| M | T | W | T | F | S | S |

BACK ☐ BICEPS ☐ LEGS ☐ ABS ☐
CHEST ☐ TRICEPS ☐ CALVES ☐ OTHER ☐
CARDIO ☐ FOREARMS ☐ SHOULDERS ☐

EXERCISE

1 234567   WEIGHT | REPS | REPS | REPS | REPS | REPS | REPS |

EXERCISE

1 **2** 34567   WEIGHT | REPS | REPS | REPS | REPS | REPS | REPS |

EXERCISE

12 **3** 4567   WEIGHT | REPS | REPS | REPS | REPS | REPS | REPS |

EXERCISE

123 **4** 567   WEIGHT | REPS | REPS | REPS | REPS | REPS | REPS |

EXERCISE

1234 **5** 67   WEIGHT | REPS | REPS | REPS | REPS | REPS | REPS |

EXERCISE

12345 **6** 7   WEIGHT | REPS | REPS | REPS | REPS | REPS | REPS |

EXERCISE

123456 **7**   WEIGHT | REPS | REPS | REPS | REPS | REPS | REPS |

CARDIO | TIME | DIST. | PACE | INT. | HR |

PRE-WORKOUT

POST-WORKOUT

DATE: TIME:

M **T** **W** **T** **F** **S** **S**

BACK ☐ BICEPS ☐ LEGS ☐ ABS ☐
CHEST ☐ TRICEPS ☐ CALVES ☐ OTHER ☐
CARDIO ☐ FOREARMS ☐ SHOULDERS ☐

EXERCISE	REPS	REPS	REPS	REPS	REPS	REPS
1 2 3 4 5 6 7 WEIGHT						

EXERCISE	REPS	REPS	REPS	REPS	REPS	REPS
1 **2** 3 4 5 6 7 WEIGHT						

EXERCISE	REPS	REPS	REPS	REPS	REPS	REPS
1 2 **3** 4 5 6 7 WEIGHT						

EXERCISE	REPS	REPS	REPS	REPS	REPS	REPS
1 2 3 **4** 5 6 7 WEIGHT						

EXERCISE	REPS	REPS	REPS	REPS	REPS	REPS
1 2 3 4 **5** 6 7 WEIGHT						

EXERCISE	REPS	REPS	REPS	REPS	REPS	REPS
1 2 3 4 5 **6** 7 WEIGHT						

EXERCISE	REPS	REPS	REPS	REPS	REPS	REPS
1 2 3 4 5 6 **7** WEIGHT						

CARDIO	TIME	DIST.	PACE	INT.	HR	
PRE-WORKOUT						
POST-WORKOUT						

DATE: TIME:

M T W T F S S

BACK ☐   BICEPS ☐   LEGS ☐   ABS ☐
CHEST ☐   TRICEPS ☐   CALVES ☐   OTHER ☐
CARDIO ☐   FOREARMS ☐   SHOULDERS ☐

EXERCISE   REPS   REPS   REPS   REPS   REPS   REPS

1 234567   WEIGHT

EXERCISE   REPS   REPS   REPS   REPS   REPS   REPS

1 **2** 34567   WEIGHT

EXERCISE   REPS   REPS   REPS   REPS   REPS   REPS

12 **3** 4567   WEIGHT

EXERCISE   REPS   REPS   REPS   REPS   REPS   REPS

123 **4** 567   WEIGHT

EXERCISE   REPS   REPS   REPS   REPS   REPS   REPS

1234 **5** 67   WEIGHT

EXERCISE   REPS   REPS   REPS   REPS   REPS   REPS

12345 **6** 7   WEIGHT

EXERCISE   REPS   REPS   REPS   REPS   REPS   REPS

123456 **7**   WEIGHT

CARDIO   TIME   DIST.   PACE   INT.   HR

PRE-WORKOUT

POST-WORKOUT

DATE:
TIME:
M T W T F S S
BACK
CHEST
CARDIO
BICEPS
TRICEPS
FOREARMS
LEGS
CALVES
SHOULDERS
ABS
OTHER

EXERCISE
REPS REPS REPS REPS REPS REPS
1 234567
WEIGHT

EXERCISE
REPS REPS REPS REPS REPS REPS
1 2 34567
WEIGHT

EXERCISE
REPS REPS REPS REPS REPS REPS
12 3 4567
WEIGHT

EXERCISE
REPS REPS REPS REPS REPS REPS
123 4 567
WEIGHT

EXERCISE
REPS REPS REPS REPS REPS REPS
1234 5 67
WEIGHT

EXERCISE
REPS REPS REPS REPS REPS REPS
12345 6 7
WEIGHT

EXERCISE
REPS REPS REPS REPS REPS REPS
123456 7
WEIGHT

CARDIO
TIME DIST. PACE INT. HR
PRE-WORKOUT
POST-WORKOUT

DATE:
TIME:
M T W T F S S
BACK ☐ BICEPS ☐ LEGS ☐ ABS ☐
CHEST ☐ TRICEPS ☐ CALVES ☐ OTHER ☐
CARDIO ☐ FOREARMS ☐ SHOULDERS ☐
EXERCISE
REPS REPS REPS REPS REPS REPS
1 234567 WEIGHT
EXERCISE
REPS REPS REPS REPS REPS REPS
1 2 34567 WEIGHT
EXERCISE
REPS REPS REPS REPS REPS REPS
12 3 4567 WEIGHT
EXERCISE
REPS REPS REPS REPS REPS REPS
123 4 567 WEIGHT
EXERCISE
REPS REPS REPS REPS REPS REPS
1234 5 67 WEIGHT
EXERCISE
REPS REPS REPS REPS REPS REPS
12345 6 7 WEIGHT
EXERCISE
REPS REPS REPS REPS REPS REPS
123456 7 WEIGHT
CARDIO TIME DIST. PACE INT. HR
PRE-WORKOUT
POST-WORKOUT

DATE: TIME:

M **T** **W** **T** **F** **S** **S**

BACK ☐   BICEPS ☐   LEGS ☐   ABS ☐
CHEST ☐   TRICEPS ☐   CALVES ☐   OTHER ☐
CARDIO ☐   FOREARMS ☐   SHOULDERS ☐

EXERCISE	REPS	REPS	REPS	REPS	REPS	REPS
1 234567 WEIGHT						

EXERCISE	REPS	REPS	REPS	REPS	REPS	REPS
1 **2** 34567 WEIGHT						

EXERCISE	REPS	REPS	REPS	REPS	REPS	REPS
12 **3** 4567 WEIGHT						

EXERCISE	REPS	REPS	REPS	REPS	REPS	REPS
123 **4** 567 WEIGHT						

EXERCISE	REPS	REPS	REPS	REPS	REPS	REPS
1234 **5** 67 WEIGHT						

EXERCISE	REPS	REPS	REPS	REPS	REPS	REPS
12345 **6** 7 WEIGHT						

EXERCISE	REPS	REPS	REPS	REPS	REPS	REPS
123456 **7** WEIGHT						

CARDIO	TIME	DIST.	PACE	INT.	HR	
PRE-WORKOUT						
POST-WORKOUT						

DATE: | TIME:

M **T** **W** **T** **F** **S** **S**

BACK ☐   BICEPS ☐   LEGS ☐   ABS ☐
CHEST ☐   TRICEPS ☐   CALVES ☐   OTHER ☐
CARDIO ☐   FOREARMS ☐   SHOULDERS ☐

EXERCISE

REPS	REPS	REPS	REPS	REPS	REPS

1 2 3 4 5 6 7   WEIGHT

EXERCISE

REPS	REPS	REPS	REPS	REPS	REPS

1 **2** 3 4 5 6 7   WEIGHT

EXERCISE

REPS	REPS	REPS	REPS	REPS	REPS

1 2 **3** 4 5 6 7   WEIGHT

EXERCISE

REPS	REPS	REPS	REPS	REPS	REPS

1 2 3 **4** 5 6 7   WEIGHT

EXERCISE

REPS	REPS	REPS	REPS	REPS	REPS

1 2 3 4 **5** 6 7   WEIGHT

EXERCISE

REPS	REPS	REPS	REPS	REPS	REPS

1 2 3 4 5 **6** 7   WEIGHT

EXERCISE

REPS	REPS	REPS	REPS	REPS	REPS

1 2 3 4 5 6 **7**   WEIGHT

CARDIO

	TIME	DIST.	PACE	INT.	HR
PRE-WORKOUT					
POST-WORKOUT					

EXERCISE	REPS	REPS	REPS	REPS	REPS	REPS
1 2 3 4 5 6 7 WEIGHT						

EXERCISE	REPS	REPS	REPS	REPS	REPS	REPS
1 **2** 3 4 5 6 7 WEIGHT						

EXERCISE	REPS	REPS	REPS	REPS	REPS	REPS
1 2 **3** 4 5 6 7 WEIGHT						

EXERCISE	REPS	REPS	REPS	REPS	REPS	REPS
1 2 3 **4** 5 6 7 WEIGHT						

EXERCISE	REPS	REPS	REPS	REPS	REPS	REPS
1 2 3 4 **5** 6 7 WEIGHT						

EXERCISE	REPS	REPS	REPS	REPS	REPS	REPS
1 2 3 4 5 **6** 7 WEIGHT						

EXERCISE	REPS	REPS	REPS	REPS	REPS	REPS
1 2 3 4 5 6 **7** WEIGHT						

CARDIO	TIME	DIST.	PACE	INT.	HR
PRE-WORKOUT					
POST-WORKOUT					

DATE:
TIME:
M T W T F S S
BACK ☐ BICEPS ☐ LEGS ☐ ABS ☐
CHEST ☐ TRICEPS ☐ CALVES ☐ OTHER ☐
CARDIO ☐ FOREARMS ☐ SHOULDERS ☐

EXERCISE
REPS REPS REPS REPS REPS REPS
1 234567 WEIGHT

EXERCISE
REPS REPS REPS REPS REPS REPS
1 2 34567 WEIGHT

EXERCISE
REPS REPS REPS REPS REPS REPS
12 3 4567 WEIGHT

EXERCISE
REPS REPS REPS REPS REPS REPS
123 4 567 WEIGHT

EXERCISE
REPS REPS REPS REPS REPS REPS
1234 5 67 WEIGHT

EXERCISE
REPS REPS REPS REPS REPS REPS
12345 6 7 WEIGHT

EXERCISE
REPS REPS REPS REPS REPS REPS
123456 7 WEIGHT

CARDIO   TIME   DIST.   PACE   INT.   HR
PRE-WORKOUT
POST-WORKOUT

DATE: TIME:

M **T** **W** **T** **F** **S** **S**

BACK ☐   BICEPS ☐   LEGS ☐   ABS ☐
CHEST ☐   TRICEPS ☐   CALVES ☐   OTHER ☐
CARDIO ☐   FOREARMS ☐   SHOULDERS ☐

EXERCISE	REPS	REPS	REPS	REPS	REPS	REPS
1 2 3 4 5 6 7 — WEIGHT						
EXERCISE — REPS ×6						
1 **2** 3 4 5 6 7 — WEIGHT						
EXERCISE — REPS ×6						
1 2 **3** 4 5 6 7 — WEIGHT						
EXERCISE — REPS ×6						
1 2 3 **4** 5 6 7 — WEIGHT						
EXERCISE — REPS ×6						
1 2 3 4 **5** 6 7 — WEIGHT						
EXERCISE — REPS ×6						
1 2 3 4 5 **6** 7 — WEIGHT						
EXERCISE — REPS ×6						
1 2 3 4 5 6 **7** — WEIGHT						

CARDIO	TIME	DIST.	PACE	INT.	HR	
PRE-WORKOUT						
POST-WORKOUT						

DATE: TIME:

M T W T F S S

BACK ☐   BICEPS ☐   LEGS ☐   ABS ☐
CHEST ☐   TRICEPS ☐   CALVES ☐   OTHER ☐
CARDIO ☐   FOREARMS ☐   SHOULDERS ☐

EXERCISE

REPS   **REPS**   **REPS**   **REPS**   **REPS**   **REPS**

1 2 3 4 5 6 7   WEIGHT

EXERCISE

REPS   **REPS**   **REPS**   **REPS**   **REPS**   **REPS**

1 **2** 3 4 5 6 7   WEIGHT

EXERCISE

REPS   **REPS**   **REPS**   **REPS**   **REPS**   **REPS**

1 2 **3** 4 5 6 7   WEIGHT

EXERCISE

REPS   **REPS**   **REPS**   **REPS**   **REPS**   **REPS**

1 2 3 **4** 5 6 7   WEIGHT

EXERCISE

REPS   **REPS**   **REPS**   **REPS**   **REPS**   **REPS**

1 2 3 4 **5** 6 7   WEIGHT

EXERCISE

REPS   **REPS**   **REPS**   **REPS**   **REPS**   **REPS**

1 2 3 4 5 **6** 7   WEIGHT

EXERCISE

REPS   **REPS**   **REPS**   **REPS**   **REPS**   **REPS**

1 2 3 4 5 6 **7**   WEIGHT

CARDIO

	TIME	DIST.	PACE	INT.	HR
PRE-WORKOUT					
POST-WORKOUT					

DATE: | TIME:

M T W T F S S

BACK ☐   BICEPS ☐   LEGS ☐   ABS ☐
CHEST ☐   TRICEPS ☐   CALVES ☐   OTHER ☐
CARDIO ☐   FOREARMS ☐   SHOULDERS ☐

EXERCISE	REPS	REPS	REPS	REPS	REPS	REPS
1 2 3 4 5 6 7 WEIGHT						
EXERCISE	REPS	REPS	REPS	REPS	REPS	REPS
1 **2** 3 4 5 6 7 WEIGHT						
EXERCISE	REPS	REPS	REPS	REPS	REPS	REPS
1 2 **3** 4 5 6 7 WEIGHT						
EXERCISE	REPS	REPS	REPS	REPS	REPS	REPS
1 2 3 **4** 5 6 7 WEIGHT						
EXERCISE	REPS	REPS	REPS	REPS	REPS	REPS
1 2 3 4 **5** 6 7 WEIGHT						
EXERCISE	REPS	REPS	REPS	REPS	REPS	REPS
1 2 3 4 5 **6** 7 WEIGHT						
EXERCISE	REPS	REPS	REPS	REPS	REPS	REPS
1 2 3 4 5 6 **7** WEIGHT						

CARDIO	TIME	DIST.	PACE	INT.	HR	
PRE-WORKOUT						
POST-WORKOUT						

DATE:	TIME:

M **T** **W** **T** **F** **S** **S**

BACK ☐ BICEPS ☐ LEGS ☐ ABS ☐
CHEST ☐ TRICEPS ☐ CALVES ☐ OTHER ☐
CARDIO ☐ FOREARMS ☐ SHOULDERS ☐

EXERCISE

1 2 3 4 5 6 7   WEIGHT

REPS	REPS	REPS	REPS	REPS	REPS

EXERCISE

1 **2** 3 4 5 6 7   WEIGHT

REPS	REPS	REPS	REPS	REPS	REPS

EXERCISE

1 2 **3** 4 5 6 7   WEIGHT

REPS	REPS	REPS	REPS	REPS	REPS

EXERCISE

1 2 3 **4** 5 6 7   WEIGHT

REPS	REPS	REPS	REPS	REPS	REPS

EXERCISE

1 2 3 4 **5** 6 7   WEIGHT

REPS	REPS	REPS	REPS	REPS	REPS

EXERCISE

1 2 3 4 5 **6** 7   WEIGHT

REPS	REPS	REPS	REPS	REPS	REPS

EXERCISE

1 2 3 4 5 6 **7**   WEIGHT

REPS	REPS	REPS	REPS	REPS	REPS

CARDIO	TIME	DIST.	PACE	INT.	HR	
PRE-WORKOUT						
POST-WORKOUT						

DATE: TIME:

M T W T F S S

BACK ☐ BICEPS ☐ LEGS ☐ ABS ☐
CHEST ☐ TRICEPS ☐ CALVES ☐ OTHER ☐
CARDIO ☐ FOREARMS ☐ SHOULDERS ☐

EXERCISE	REPS	REPS	REPS	REPS	REPS	REPS
1 2 3 4 5 6 7 — WEIGHT						
2 — WEIGHT (1 **2** 3 4 5 6 7)						
1 2 **3** 4 5 6 7 — WEIGHT						
1 2 3 **4** 5 6 7 — WEIGHT						
1 2 3 4 **5** 6 7 — WEIGHT						
1 2 3 4 5 **6** 7 — WEIGHT						
1 2 3 4 5 6 **7** — WEIGHT						

CARDIO	TIME	DIST.	PACE	INT.	HR	
PRE-WORKOUT						
POST-WORKOUT						

DATE: TIME: BACK ☐ BICEPS ☐ LEGS ☐ ABS ☐

M T W T F S S   CHEST ☐ TRICEPS ☐ CALVES ☐ OTHER ☐

CARDIO ☐ FOREARMS ☐ SHOULDERS ☐

EXERCISE

	REPS	REPS	REPS	REPS	REPS	REPS
1 234567 WEIGHT						

EXERCISE

	REPS	REPS	REPS	REPS	REPS	REPS
1 **2** 34567 WEIGHT						

EXERCISE

	REPS	REPS	REPS	REPS	REPS	REPS
12 **3** 4567 WEIGHT						

EXERCISE

	REPS	REPS	REPS	REPS	REPS	REPS
123 **4** 567 WEIGHT						

EXERCISE

	REPS	REPS	REPS	REPS	REPS	REPS
1234 **5** 67 WEIGHT						

EXERCISE

	REPS	REPS	REPS	REPS	REPS	REPS
12345 **6** 7 WEIGHT						

EXERCISE

	REPS	REPS	REPS	REPS	REPS	REPS
123456 **7** WEIGHT						

CARDIO

	TIME	DIST.	PACE	INT.	HR	
PRE-WORKOUT						
POST-WORKOUT						

DATE: TIME:

M T W T F S S

BACK ☐   BICEPS ☐   LEGS ☐   ABS ☐
CHEST ☐   TRICEPS ☐   CALVES ☐   OTHER ☐
CARDIO ☐   FOREARMS ☐   SHOULDERS ☐

EXERCISE	REPS	REPS	REPS	REPS	REPS	REPS
1 234567 WEIGHT						
1**2**34567 WEIGHT						
12**3**4567 WEIGHT						
123**4**567 WEIGHT						
1234**5**67 WEIGHT						
12345**6**7 WEIGHT						
123456**7** WEIGHT						

CARDIO	TIME	DIST.	PACE	INT.	HR
PRE-WORKOUT					
POST-WORKOUT					

| DATE: | TIME: |

M T W T F S S

BACK ☐ BICEPS ☐ LEGS ☐ ABS ☐
CHEST ☐ TRICEPS ☐ CALVES ☐ OTHER ☐
CARDIO ☐ FOREARMS ☐ SHOULDERS ☐

EXERCISE

1 2 3 4 5 6 7   WEIGHT

REPS	REPS	REPS	REPS	REPS	REPS

EXERCISE

1 **2** 3 4 5 6 7   WEIGHT

REPS	REPS	REPS	REPS	REPS	REPS

EXERCISE

1 2 **3** 4 5 6 7   WEIGHT

REPS	REPS	REPS	REPS	REPS	REPS

EXERCISE

1 2 3 **4** 5 6 7   WEIGHT

REPS	REPS	REPS	REPS	REPS	REPS

EXERCISE

1 2 3 4 **5** 6 7   WEIGHT

REPS	REPS	REPS	REPS	REPS	REPS

EXERCISE

1 2 3 4 5 **6** 7   WEIGHT

REPS	REPS	REPS	REPS	REPS	REPS

EXERCISE

1 2 3 4 5 6 **7**   WEIGHT

REPS	REPS	REPS	REPS	REPS	REPS

CARDIO	TIME	DIST.	PACE	INT.	HR
PRE-WORKOUT					
POST-WORKOUT					

DATE:	TIME:	BACK ☐	BICEPS ☐	LEGS ☐	ABS ☐
CHEST ☐	TRICEPS ☐	CALVES ☐	OTHER ☐
M	T	W	T	F	S	S	CARDIO ☐	FOREARMS ☐	SHOULDERS ☐

EXERCISE

1 2 3 4 5 6 7 — WEIGHT

| REPS ☐ | REPS ☐ | REPS ☐ | REPS ☐ | REPS ☐ | REPS ☐ |

EXERCISE

1 **2** 3 4 5 6 7 — WEIGHT

| REPS ☐ | REPS ☐ | REPS ☐ | REPS ☐ | REPS ☐ | REPS ☐ |

EXERCISE

1 2 **3** 4 5 6 7 — WEIGHT

| REPS ☐ | REPS ☐ | REPS ☐ | REPS ☐ | REPS ☐ | REPS ☐ |

EXERCISE

1 2 3 **4** 5 6 7 — WEIGHT

| REPS ☐ | REPS ☐ | REPS ☐ | REPS ☐ | REPS ☐ | REPS ☐ |

EXERCISE

1 2 3 4 **5** 6 7 — WEIGHT

| REPS ☐ | REPS ☐ | REPS ☐ | REPS ☐ | REPS ☐ | REPS ☐ |

EXERCISE

1 2 3 4 5 **6** 7 — WEIGHT

| REPS ☐ | REPS ☐ | REPS ☐ | REPS ☐ | REPS ☐ | REPS ☐ |

EXERCISE

1 2 3 4 5 6 **7** — WEIGHT

| REPS | REPS | REPS | REPS | REPS | REPS |

CARDIO

	TIME	DIST.	PACE	INT.	HR
PRE-WORKOUT					
POST-WORKOUT					

DATE:
TIME:
M T W T F S S

BACK ☐ BICEPS ☐ LEGS ☐ ABS ☐
CHEST ☐ TRICEPS ☐ CALVES ☐ OTHER ☐
CARDIO ☐ FOREARMS ☐ SHOULDERS ☐

EXERCISE
REPS REPS REPS REPS REPS REPS
1 234567   WEIGHT

EXERCISE
REPS REPS REPS REPS REPS REPS
1 2 34567   WEIGHT

EXERCISE
REPS REPS REPS REPS REPS REPS
12 3 4567   WEIGHT

EXERCISE
REPS REPS REPS REPS REPS REPS
123 4 567   WEIGHT

EXERCISE
REPS REPS REPS REPS REPS REPS
1234 5 67   WEIGHT

EXERCISE
REPS REPS REPS REPS REPS REPS
12345 6 7   WEIGHT

EXERCISE
REPS REPS REPS REPS REPS REPS
123456 7   WEIGHT

CARDIO   TIME DIST. PACE INT. HR
PRE-WORKOUT
POST-WORKOUT

DATE: TIME:

M T W T F S S

BACK ☐	BICEPS ☐	LEGS ☐	ABS ☐
CHEST ☐	TRICEPS ☐	CALVES ☐	OTHER ☐
CARDIO ☐	FOREARMS ☐	SHOULDERS ☐	

EXERCISE

1 234567   WEIGHT

REPS REPS REPS REPS REPS REPS

EXERCISE

1 **2** 34567   WEIGHT

REPS REPS REPS REPS REPS REPS

EXERCISE

12 **3** 4567   WEIGHT

REPS REPS REPS REPS REPS REPS

EXERCISE

123 **4** 567   WEIGHT

REPS REPS REPS REPS REPS REPS

EXERCISE

1234 **5** 67   WEIGHT

REPS REPS REPS REPS REPS REPS

EXERCISE

12345 **6** 7   WEIGHT

REPS REPS REPS REPS REPS REPS

EXERCISE

123456 **7**   WEIGHT

REPS REPS REPS REPS REPS REPS

CARDIO

	TIME	DIST.	PACE	INT.	HR
PRE-WORKOUT					
POST-WORKOUT					

| DATE: | TIME: |

M T W T F S S

BACK ☐   BICEPS ☐   LEGS ☐   ABS ☐
CHEST ☐   TRICEPS ☐   CALVES ☐   OTHER ☐
CARDIO ☐   FOREARMS ☐   SHOULDERS ☐

EXERCISE | REPS | REPS | REPS | REPS | REPS | REPS
1 2 3 4 5 6 7   WEIGHT

EXERCISE | REPS | REPS | REPS | REPS | REPS | REPS
1 **2** 3 4 5 6 7   WEIGHT

EXERCISE | REPS | REPS | REPS | REPS | REPS | REPS
1 2 **3** 4 5 6 7   WEIGHT

EXERCISE | REPS | REPS | REPS | REPS | REPS | REPS
1 2 3 **4** 5 6 7   WEIGHT

EXERCISE | REPS | REPS | REPS | REPS | REPS | REPS
1 2 3 4 **5** 6 7   WEIGHT

EXERCISE | REPS | REPS | REPS | REPS | REPS | REPS
1 2 3 4 5 **6** 7   WEIGHT

EXERCISE | REPS | REPS | REPS | REPS | REPS | REPS
1 2 3 4 5 6 **7**   WEIGHT

CARDIO	TIME	DIST.	PACE	INT.	HR
PRE-WORKOUT					
POST-WORKOUT					

Monthly Planner

Month: _________ Year: _________

Monday	Tuesday	Wednesday	Thursday	Friday	Saturday	Sunday
☐	☐	☐	☐	☐	☐	☐
☐	☐	☐	☐	☐	☐	☐
☐	☐	☐	☐	☐	☐	☐
☐	☐	☐	☐	☐	☐	☐
☐	☐	☐	☐	☐	☐	☐

Notes:
____
____
____
____
____
____
____
____
____

BODY PROGRESS TRACKER

WAIST

Week 1: _______________

Week 2: _______________

Week 3: _______________

Week 4: _______________

ARMS

Week 1: _______________

Week 2: _______________

Week 3: _______________

Week 4: _______________

THIGHS

Week 1: _______________

Week 2: _______________

Week 3: _______________

Week 4: _______________

HIPS

Week 1: _______________

Week 2: _______________

Week 3: _______________

Week 4: _______________

Goal Tracker	Week 1:	Week 2:	Week 3:	Week 4:
DATE				
ARMS				
WAIST				
HIPS				
THIGHS				
WEIGHT				

Weekly Meal Planner

Monday

Tuesday

Wednesday

Thursday

Friday

Saturday

Sunday

Shopping List

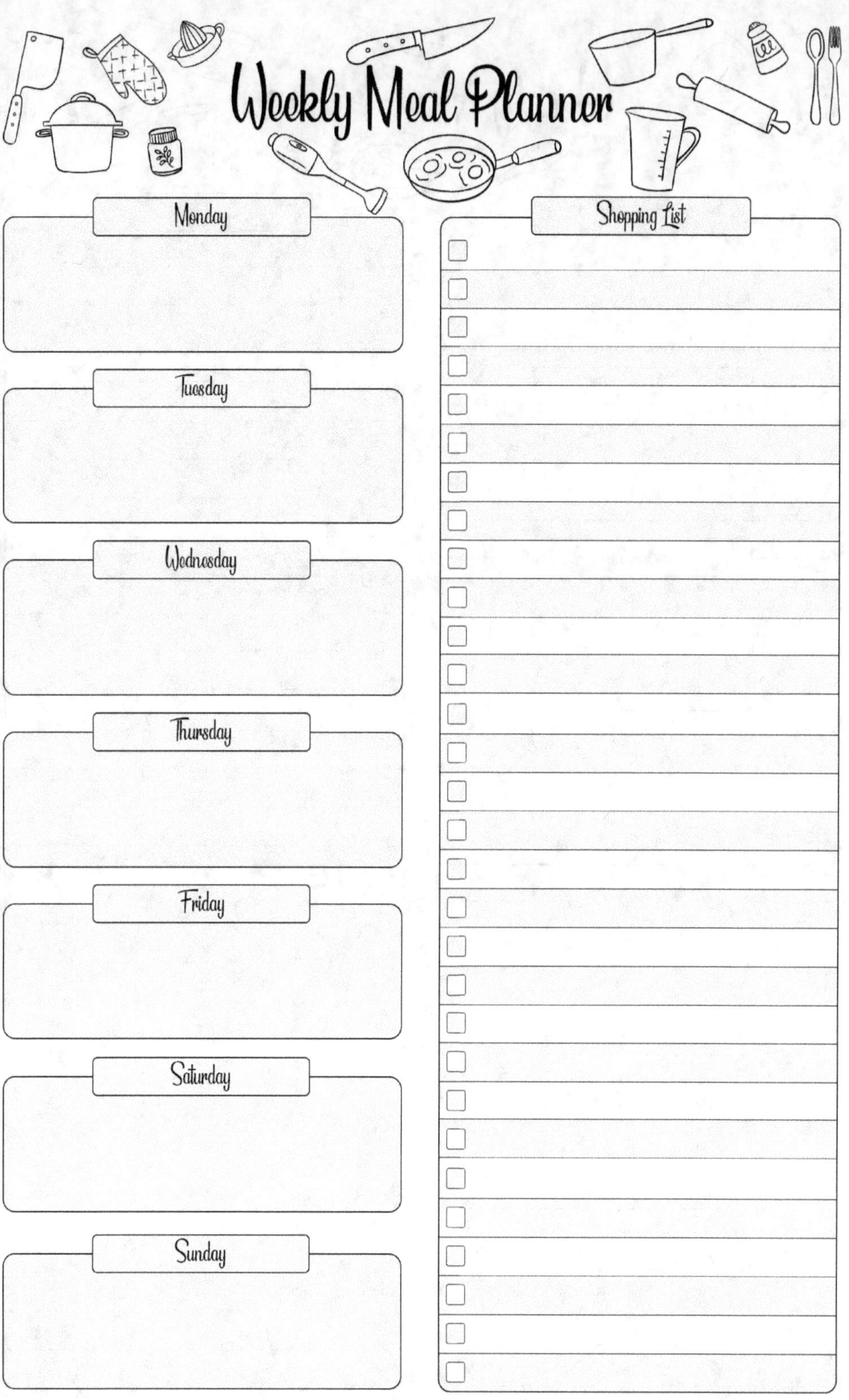
Weekly Meal Planner
Monday
Tuesday
Wednesday
Thursday
Friday
Saturday
Sunday
Shopping List

Weekly Meal Planner

Monday

Tuesday

Wednesday

Thursday

Friday

Saturday

Sunday

Shopping List

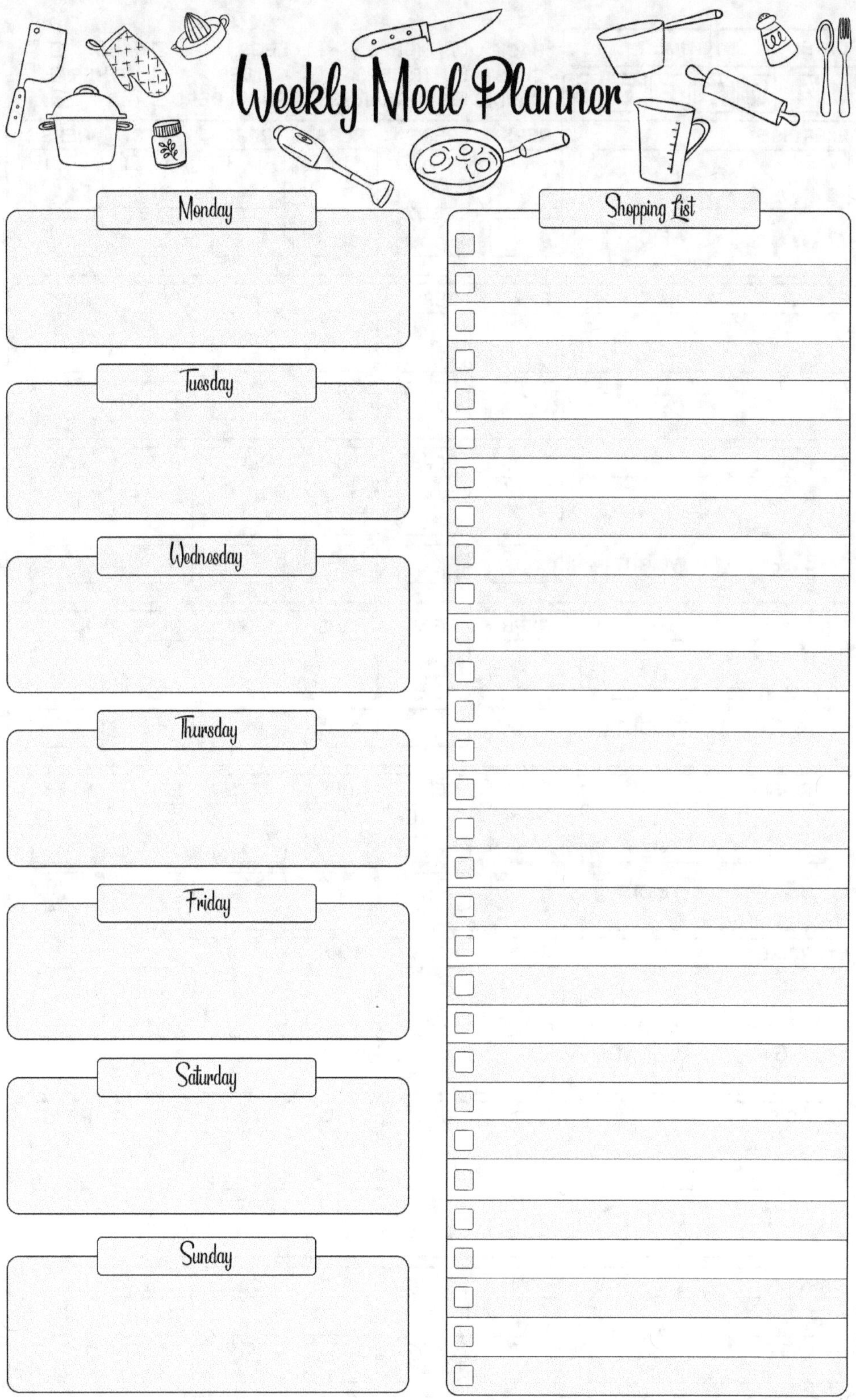# Weekly Meal Planner

| DATE: | TIME: |

M T W T F S S

BACK ☐ BICEPS ☐ LEGS ☐ ABS ☐
CHEST ☐ TRICEPS ☐ CALVES ☐ OTHER ☐
CARDIO ☐ FOREARMS ☐ SHOULDERS ☐

EXERCISE — **1** 234567 — WEIGHT — REPS | REPS | REPS | REPS | REPS | REPS

EXERCISE — 1 **2** 34567 — WEIGHT — REPS | REPS | REPS | REPS | REPS | REPS

EXERCISE — 12 **3** 4567 — WEIGHT — REPS | REPS | REPS | REPS | REPS | REPS

EXERCISE — 123 **4** 567 — WEIGHT — REPS | REPS | REPS | REPS | REPS | REPS

EXERCISE — 1234 **5** 67 — WEIGHT — REPS | REPS | REPS | REPS | REPS | REPS

EXERCISE — 12345 **6** 7 — WEIGHT — REPS | REPS | REPS | REPS | REPS | REPS

EXERCISE — 123456 **7** — WEIGHT — REPS | REPS | REPS | REPS | REPS | REPS

CARDIO | TIME | DIST. | PACE | INT. | HR

PRE-WORKOUT

POST-WORKOUT

DATE: | TIME:

M **T** **W** **T** **F** **S** **S**

BACK ☐   BICEPS ☐   LEGS ☐   ABS ☐
CHEST ☐   TRICEPS ☐   CALVES ☐   OTHER ☐
CARDIO ☐   FOREARMS ☐   SHOULDERS ☐

EXERCISE

REPS	REPS	REPS	REPS	REPS	REPS
☐	☐	☐	☐	☐	☐

1 2 3 4 5 6 7   WEIGHT

EXERCISE

REPS	REPS	REPS	REPS	REPS	REPS
☐	☐	☐	☐	☐	☐

1 **2** 3 4 5 6 7   WEIGHT

EXERCISE

REPS	REPS	REPS	REPS	REPS	REPS
☐	☐	☐	☐	☐	☐

1 2 **3** 4 5 6 7   WEIGHT

EXERCISE

REPS	REPS	REPS	REPS	REPS	REPS
☐	☐	☐	☐	☐	☐

1 2 3 **4** 5 6 7   WEIGHT

EXERCISE

REPS	REPS	REPS	REPS	REPS	REPS
☐	☐	☐	☐	☐	☐

1 2 3 4 **5** 6 7   WEIGHT

EXERCISE

REPS	REPS	REPS	REPS	REPS	REPS
☐	☐	☐	☐	☐	☐

1 2 3 4 5 **6** 7   WEIGHT

EXERCISE

REPS	REPS	REPS	REPS	REPS	REPS
☐	☐	☐	☐	☐	☐

1 2 3 4 5 6 **7**   WEIGHT

CARDIO

	TIME	DIST.	PACE	INT.	HR
PRE-WORKOUT					
POST-WORKOUT					

DATE: TIME:

M T W T F S S

BACK ☐   BICEPS ☐   LEGS ☐   ABS ☐
CHEST ☐   TRICEPS ☐   CALVES ☐   OTHER ☐
CARDIO ☐   FOREARMS ☐   SHOULDERS ☐

EXERCISE	REPS	REPS	REPS	REPS	REPS	REPS
1 234567 WEIGHT						

EXERCISE	REPS	REPS	REPS	REPS	REPS	REPS
1 **2** 34567 WEIGHT						

EXERCISE	REPS	REPS	REPS	REPS	REPS	REPS
12 **3** 4567 WEIGHT						

EXERCISE	REPS	REPS	REPS	REPS	REPS	REPS
123 **4** 567 WEIGHT						

EXERCISE	REPS	REPS	REPS	REPS	REPS	REPS
1234 **5** 67 WEIGHT						

EXERCISE	REPS	REPS	REPS	REPS	REPS	REPS
12345 **6** 7 WEIGHT						

EXERCISE	REPS	REPS	REPS	REPS	REPS	REPS
123456 **7** WEIGHT						

CARDIO	TIME	DIST.	PACE	INT.	HR	
PRE-WORKOUT						
POST-WORKOUT						

DATE: TIME:

M **T** **W** **T** **F** **S** **S**

BACK ☐   BICEPS ☐   LEGS ☐   ABS ☐
CHEST ☐   TRICEPS ☐   CALVES ☐   OTHER ☐
CARDIO ☐   FOREARMS ☐   SHOULDERS ☐

EXERCISE	REPS	REPS	REPS	REPS	REPS	REPS
1 234567 WEIGHT						

EXERCISE	REPS	REPS	REPS	REPS	REPS	REPS
1 **2** 34567 WEIGHT						

EXERCISE	REPS	REPS	REPS	REPS	REPS	REPS
12 **3** 4567 WEIGHT						

EXERCISE	REPS	REPS	REPS	REPS	REPS	REPS
123 **4** 567 WEIGHT						

EXERCISE	REPS	REPS	REPS	REPS	REPS	REPS
1234 **5** 67 WEIGHT						

EXERCISE	REPS	REPS	REPS	REPS	REPS	REPS
12345 **6** 7 WEIGHT						

EXERCISE	REPS	REPS	REPS	REPS	REPS	REPS
123456 **7** WEIGHT						

CARDIO	TIME	DIST.	PACE	INT.	HR	
PRE-WORKOUT						
POST-WORKOUT						

DATE: TIME:

M T W T F S S

BACK ☐ BICEPS ☐ LEGS ☐ ABS ☐
CHEST ☐ TRICEPS ☐ CALVES ☐ OTHER ☐
CARDIO ☐ FOREARMS ☐ SHOULDERS ☐

EXERCISE REPS REPS REPS REPS REPS REPS
1 234567 WEIGHT

EXERCISE REPS REPS REPS REPS REPS REPS
1 **2** 34567 WEIGHT

EXERCISE REPS REPS REPS REPS REPS REPS
12 **3** 4567 WEIGHT

EXERCISE REPS REPS REPS REPS REPS REPS
123 **4** 567 WEIGHT

EXERCISE REPS REPS REPS REPS REPS REPS
1234 **5** 67 WEIGHT

EXERCISE REPS REPS REPS REPS REPS REPS
12345 **6** 7 WEIGHT

EXERCISE REPS REPS REPS REPS REPS REPS
123456 **7** WEIGHT

CARDIO TIME DIST. PACE INT. HR
PRE-WORKOUT
POST-WORKOUT

DATE: TIME:

M **T** **W** **T** **F** **S** **S**

BACK ☐   BICEPS ☐   LEGS ☐   ABS ☐
CHEST ☐   TRICEPS ☐   CALVES ☐   OTHER ☐
CARDIO ☐   FOREARMS ☐   SHOULDERS ☐

EXERCISE

REPS   REPS   REPS   REPS   REPS   REPS

1 2 3 4 5 6 7   WEIGHT

EXERCISE

REPS   REPS   REPS   REPS   REPS   REPS

1 **2** 3 4 5 6 7   WEIGHT

EXERCISE

REPS   REPS   REPS   REPS   REPS   REPS

1 2 **3** 4 5 6 7   WEIGHT

EXERCISE

REPS   REPS   REPS   REPS   REPS   REPS

1 2 3 **4** 5 6 7   WEIGHT

EXERCISE

REPS   REPS   REPS   REPS   REPS   REPS

1 2 3 4 **5** 6 7   WEIGHT

EXERCISE

REPS   REPS   REPS   REPS   REPS   REPS

1 2 3 4 5 **6** 7   WEIGHT

EXERCISE

REPS   REPS   REPS   REPS   REPS   REPS

1 2 3 4 5 6 **7**   WEIGHT

CARDIO

TIME   DIST.   PACE   INT.   HR

PRE-WORKOUT

POST-WORKOUT

DATE: TIME:

M **T** **W** **T** **F** **S** **S**

BACK ☐   BICEPS ☐   LEGS ☐   ABS ☐
CHEST ☐   TRICEPS ☐   CALVES ☐   OTHER ☐
CARDIO ☐   FOREARMS ☐   SHOULDERS ☐

EXERCISE	REPS	REPS	REPS	REPS	REPS	REPS
1 234567 WEIGHT						

EXERCISE	REPS	REPS	REPS	REPS	REPS	REPS
1 **2** 34567 WEIGHT						

EXERCISE	REPS	REPS	REPS	REPS	REPS	REPS
12 **3** 4567 WEIGHT						

EXERCISE	REPS	REPS	REPS	REPS	REPS	REPS
123 **4** 567 WEIGHT						

EXERCISE	REPS	REPS	REPS	REPS	REPS	REPS
1234 **5** 67 WEIGHT						

EXERCISE	REPS	REPS	REPS	REPS	REPS	REPS
12345 **6** 7 WEIGHT						

EXERCISE	REPS	REPS	REPS	REPS	REPS	REPS
123456 **7** WEIGHT						

CARDIO	TIME	DIST.	PACE	INT.	HR	
PRE-WORKOUT						
POST-WORKOUT						

DATE: | TIME:

M **T** **W** **T** **F** **S** **S**

BACK ☐ BICEPS ☐ LEGS ☐ ABS ☐
CHEST ☐ TRICEPS ☐ CALVES ☐ OTHER ☐
CARDIO ☐ FOREARMS ☐ SHOULDERS ☐

EXERCISE | REPS | REPS | REPS | REPS | REPS | REPS

1 2 3 4 5 6 7 | WEIGHT

EXERCISE | REPS | REPS | REPS | REPS | REPS | REPS

1 **2** 3 4 5 6 7 | WEIGHT

EXERCISE | REPS | REPS | REPS | REPS | REPS | REPS

1 2 **3** 4 5 6 7 | WEIGHT

EXERCISE | REPS | REPS | REPS | REPS | REPS | REPS

1 2 3 **4** 5 6 7 | WEIGHT

EXERCISE | REPS | REPS | REPS | REPS | REPS | REPS

1 2 3 4 **5** 6 7 | WEIGHT

EXERCISE | REPS | REPS | REPS | REPS | REPS | REPS

1 2 3 4 5 **6** 7 | WEIGHT

EXERCISE | REPS | REPS | REPS | REPS | REPS | REPS

1 2 3 4 5 6 **7** | WEIGHT

CARDIO | TIME | DIST. | PACE | INT. | HR
PRE-WORKOUT
POST-WORKOUT

DATE: TIME:

M T W T F S S

BACK ☐ BICEPS ☐ LEGS ☐ ABS ☐
CHEST ☐ TRICEPS ☐ CALVES ☐ OTHER ☐
CARDIO ☐ FOREARMS ☐ SHOULDERS ☐

EXERCISE	REPS	REPS	REPS	REPS	REPS	REPS
1 2 3 4 5 6 7 WEIGHT						

EXERCISE	REPS	REPS	REPS	REPS	REPS	REPS
1 **2** 3 4 5 6 7 WEIGHT						

EXERCISE	REPS	REPS	REPS	REPS	REPS	REPS
1 2 **3** 4 5 6 7 WEIGHT						

EXERCISE	REPS	REPS	REPS	REPS	REPS	REPS
1 2 3 **4** 5 6 7 WEIGHT						

EXERCISE	REPS	REPS	REPS	REPS	REPS	REPS
1 2 3 4 **5** 6 7 WEIGHT						

EXERCISE	REPS	REPS	REPS	REPS	REPS	REPS
1 2 3 4 5 **6** 7 WEIGHT						

EXERCISE	REPS	REPS	REPS	REPS	REPS	REPS
1 2 3 4 5 6 **7** WEIGHT						

CARDIO	TIME	DIST.	PACE	INT.	HR	
PRE-WORKOUT						
POST-WORKOUT						

DATE: TIME:

M T W T F S S

BACK ☐   BICEPS ☐   LEGS ☐   ABS ☐
CHEST ☐   TRICEPS ☐   CALVES ☐   OTHER ☐
CARDIO ☐   FOREARMS ☐   SHOULDERS ☐

EXERCISE   REPS   REPS   REPS   REPS   REPS   REPS

1 2 3 4 5 6 7   WEIGHT

EXERCISE   REPS   REPS   REPS   REPS   REPS   REPS

1 **2** 3 4 5 6 7   WEIGHT

EXERCISE   REPS   REPS   REPS   REPS   REPS   REPS

1 2 **3** 4 5 6 7   WEIGHT

EXERCISE   REPS   REPS   REPS   REPS   REPS   REPS

1 2 3 **4** 5 6 7   WEIGHT

EXERCISE   REPS   REPS   REPS   REPS   REPS   REPS

1 2 3 4 **5** 6 7   WEIGHT

EXERCISE   REPS   REPS   REPS   REPS   REPS   REPS

1 2 3 4 5 **6** 7   WEIGHT

EXERCISE   REPS   REPS   REPS   REPS   REPS   REPS

1 2 3 4 5 6 **7**   WEIGHT

CARDIO   TIME   DIST.   PACE   INT.   HR

PRE-WORKOUT

POST-WORKOUT

DATE: TIME:

M **T** **W** **T** **F** **S** **S**

BACK ☐   BICEPS ☐   LEGS ☐   ABS ☐
CHEST ☐   TRICEPS ☐   CALVES ☐   OTHER ☐
CARDIO ☐   FOREARMS ☐   SHOULDERS ☐

EXERCISE   REPS   REPS   REPS   REPS   REPS   REPS

1 2 3 4 5 6 7   WEIGHT

EXERCISE   REPS   REPS   REPS   REPS   REPS   REPS

1 **2** 3 4 5 6 7   WEIGHT

EXERCISE   REPS   REPS   REPS   REPS   REPS   REPS

1 2 **3** 4 5 6 7   WEIGHT

EXERCISE   REPS   REPS   REPS   REPS   REPS   REPS

1 2 3 **4** 5 6 7   WEIGHT

EXERCISE   REPS   REPS   REPS   REPS   REPS   REPS

1 2 3 4 **5** 6 7   WEIGHT

EXERCISE   REPS   REPS   REPS   REPS   REPS   REPS

1 2 3 4 5 **6** 7   WEIGHT

EXERCISE   REPS   REPS   REPS   REPS   REPS   REPS

1 2 3 4 5 6 **7**   WEIGHT

CARDIO   TIME   DIST.   PACE   INT.   HR

PRE-WORKOUT

POST-WORKOUT

DATE: | TIME:

M **T** **W** **T** **F** **S** **S**

BACK ☐ BICEPS ☐ LEGS ☐ ABS ☐
CHEST ☐ TRICEPS ☐ CALVES ☐ OTHER ☐
CARDIO ☐ FOREARMS ☐ SHOULDERS ☐

EXERCISE | REPS | REPS | REPS | REPS | REPS | REPS

1 2 3 4 5 6 7 | WEIGHT

EXERCISE | REPS | REPS | REPS | REPS | REPS | REPS

1 **2** 3 4 5 6 7 | WEIGHT

EXERCISE | REPS | REPS | REPS | REPS | REPS | REPS

1 2 **3** 4 5 6 7 | WEIGHT

EXERCISE | REPS | REPS | REPS | REPS | REPS | REPS

1 2 3 **4** 5 6 7 | WEIGHT

EXERCISE | REPS | REPS | REPS | REPS | REPS | REPS

1 2 3 4 **5** 6 7 | WEIGHT

EXERCISE | REPS | REPS | REPS | REPS | REPS | REPS

1 2 3 4 5 **6** 7 | WEIGHT

EXERCISE | REPS | REPS | REPS | REPS | REPS | REPS

1 2 3 4 5 6 **7** | WEIGHT

CARDIO | TIME | DIST. | PACE | INT. | HR
PRE-WORKOUT
POST-WORKOUT

| DATE: | TIME: |

| M | T | W | T | F | S | S |

BACK ☐	BICEPS ☐	LEGS ☐	ABS ☐
CHEST ☐	TRICEPS ☐	CALVES ☐	OTHER ☐
CARDIO ☐	FOREARMS ☐	SHOULDERS ☐	

EXERCISE

	REPS	REPS	REPS	REPS	REPS	REPS
1 2 3 4 5 6 7 WEIGHT						

EXERCISE

	REPS	REPS	REPS	REPS	REPS	REPS
1 **2** 3 4 5 6 7 WEIGHT						

EXERCISE

	REPS	REPS	REPS	REPS	REPS	REPS
1 2 **3** 4 5 6 7 WEIGHT						

EXERCISE

	REPS	REPS	REPS	REPS	REPS	REPS
1 2 3 **4** 5 6 7 WEIGHT						

EXERCISE

	REPS	REPS	REPS	REPS	REPS	REPS
1 2 3 4 **5** 6 7 WEIGHT						

EXERCISE

	REPS	REPS	REPS	REPS	REPS	REPS
1 2 3 4 5 **6** 7 WEIGHT						

EXERCISE

	REPS	REPS	REPS	REPS	REPS	REPS
1 2 3 4 5 6 **7** WEIGHT						

CARDIO	TIME	DIST.	PACE	INT.	HR
PRE-WORKOUT					
POST-WORKOUT					

DATE:
TIME:
M T W T F S S
BACK ☐ BICEPS ☐ LEGS ☐ ABS ☐
CHEST ☐ TRICEPS ☐ CALVES ☐ OTHER ☐
CARDIO ☐ FOREARMS ☐ SHOULDERS ☐

EXERCISE
REPS REPS REPS REPS REPS REPS
1 234567 WEIGHT

EXERCISE
REPS REPS REPS REPS REPS REPS
1 2 34567 WEIGHT

EXERCISE
REPS REPS REPS REPS REPS REPS
12 3 4567 WEIGHT

EXERCISE
REPS REPS REPS REPS REPS REPS
123 4 567 WEIGHT

EXERCISE
REPS REPS REPS REPS REPS REPS
1234 5 67 WEIGHT

EXERCISE
REPS REPS REPS REPS REPS REPS
12345 6 7 WEIGHT

EXERCISE
REPS REPS REPS REPS REPS REPS
123456 7 WEIGHT

CARDIO
TIME DIST. PACE INT. HR
PRE-WORKOUT
POST-WORKOUT

| DATE: | TIME: |

M T W T F S S

BACK ☐	BICEPS ☐	LEGS ☐	ABS ☐
CHEST ☐	TRICEPS ☐	CALVES ☐	OTHER ☐
CARDIO ☐	FOREARMS ☐	SHOULDERS ☐	

EXERCISE · REPS · REPS · REPS · REPS · REPS · REPS
1 2 3 4 5 6 7 — WEIGHT

EXERCISE · REPS · REPS · REPS · REPS · REPS · REPS
1 **2** 3 4 5 6 7 — WEIGHT

EXERCISE · REPS · REPS · REPS · REPS · REPS · REPS
1 2 **3** 4 5 6 7 — WEIGHT

EXERCISE · REPS · REPS · REPS · REPS · REPS · REPS
1 2 3 **4** 5 6 7 — WEIGHT

EXERCISE · REPS · REPS · REPS · REPS · REPS · REPS
1 2 3 4 **5** 6 7 — WEIGHT

EXERCISE · REPS · REPS · REPS · REPS · REPS · REPS
1 2 3 4 5 **6** 7 — WEIGHT

EXERCISE · REPS · REPS · REPS · REPS · REPS · REPS
1 2 3 4 5 6 **7** — WEIGHT

CARDIO	TIME	DIST.	PACE	INT.	HR
PRE-WORKOUT					
POST-WORKOUT					

| DATE: | TIME: |

M T W T F S S

BACK ☐ BICEPS ☐ LEGS ☐ ABS ☐
CHEST ☐ TRICEPS ☐ CALVES ☐ OTHER ☐
CARDIO ☐ FOREARMS ☐ SHOULDERS ☐

EXERCISE

1 234567 WEIGHT REPS REPS REPS REPS REPS REPS

EXERCISE

1 **2** 34567 WEIGHT REPS REPS REPS REPS REPS REPS

EXERCISE

12 **3** 4567 WEIGHT REPS REPS REPS REPS REPS REPS

EXERCISE

123 **4** 567 WEIGHT REPS REPS REPS REPS REPS REPS

EXERCISE

1234 **5** 67 WEIGHT REPS REPS REPS REPS REPS REPS

EXERCISE

12345 **6** 7 WEIGHT REPS REPS REPS REPS REPS REPS

EXERCISE

123456 **7** WEIGHT REPS REPS REPS REPS REPS REPS

CARDIO | TIME | DIST. | PACE | INT. | HR

PRE-WORKOUT

POST-WORKOUT

DATE: TIME:

M T W T F S S

BACK ☐ BICEPS ☐ LEGS ☐ ABS ☐
CHEST ☐ TRICEPS ☐ CALVES ☐ OTHER ☐
CARDIO ☐ FOREARMS ☐ SHOULDERS ☐

EXERCISE
REPS REPS REPS REPS REPS REPS

1 234567 WEIGHT

EXERCISE
REPS REPS REPS REPS REPS REPS

1 **2** 34567 WEIGHT

EXERCISE
REPS REPS REPS REPS REPS REPS

12 **3** 4567 WEIGHT

EXERCISE
REPS REPS REPS REPS REPS REPS

123 **4** 567 WEIGHT

EXERCISE
REPS REPS REPS REPS REPS REPS

1234 **5** 67 WEIGHT

EXERCISE
REPS REPS REPS REPS REPS REPS

12345 **6** 7 WEIGHT

EXERCISE
REPS REPS REPS REPS REPS REPS

123456 **7** WEIGHT

CARDIO TIME DIST. PACE INT. HR

PRE-WORKOUT

POST-WORKOUT

DATE:
TIME:
M T W T F S S
BACK ☐ BICEPS ☐ LEGS ☐ ABS ☐
CHEST ☐ TRICEPS ☐ CALVES ☐ OTHER ☐
CARDIO ☐ FOREARMS ☐ SHOULDERS ☐

EXERCISE
REPS   REPS   REPS   REPS   REPS   REPS
1 234567   WEIGHT

EXERCISE
REPS   REPS   REPS   REPS   REPS   REPS
1 2 34567   WEIGHT

EXERCISE
REPS   REPS   REPS   REPS   REPS   REPS
12 3 4567   WEIGHT

EXERCISE
REPS   REPS   REPS   REPS   REPS   REPS
123 4 567   WEIGHT

EXERCISE
REPS   REPS   REPS   REPS   REPS   REPS
1234 5 67   WEIGHT

EXERCISE
REPS   REPS   REPS   REPS   REPS   REPS
12345 6 7   WEIGHT

EXERCISE
REPS   REPS   REPS   REPS   REPS   REPS
123456 7   WEIGHT

CARDIO   TIME   DIST.   PACE   INT.   HR
PRE-WORKOUT
POST-WORKOUT

DATE: TIME:

| M | T | W | T | F | S | S |

BACK ☐	BICEPS ☐	LEGS ☐	ABS ☐
CHEST ☐	TRICEPS ☐	CALVES ☐	OTHER ☐
CARDIO ☐	FOREARMS ☐	SHOULDERS ☐	

EXERCISE   REPS REPS REPS REPS REPS REPS

1 2 3 4 5 6 7   WEIGHT

EXERCISE   REPS REPS REPS REPS REPS REPS

1 **2** 3 4 5 6 7   WEIGHT

EXERCISE   REPS REPS REPS REPS REPS REPS

1 2 **3** 4 5 6 7   WEIGHT

EXERCISE   REPS REPS REPS REPS REPS REPS

1 2 3 **4** 5 6 7   WEIGHT

EXERCISE   REPS REPS REPS REPS REPS REPS

1 2 3 4 **5** 6 7   WEIGHT

EXERCISE   REPS REPS REPS REPS REPS REPS

1 2 3 4 5 **6** 7   WEIGHT

EXERCISE   REPS REPS REPS REPS REPS REPS

1 2 3 4 5 6 **7**   WEIGHT

CARDIO   TIME   DIST.   PACE   INT.   HR

PRE-WORKOUT

POST-WORKOUT

DATE:　　　TIME:

M T W T F S S

BACK ☐　BICEPS ☐　LEGS ☐　ABS ☐
CHEST ☐　TRICEPS ☐　CALVES ☐　OTHER ☐
CARDIO ☐　FOREARMS ☐　SHOULDERS ☐

EXERCISE

REPS	REPS	REPS	REPS	REPS	REPS
☐	☐	☐	☐	☐	☐

1 2 3 4 5 6 7　WEIGHT

EXERCISE

REPS	REPS	REPS	REPS	REPS	REPS
☐	☐	☐	☐	☐	☐

1 **2** 3 4 5 6 7　WEIGHT

EXERCISE

REPS	REPS	REPS	REPS	REPS	REPS
☐	☐	☐	☐	☐	☐

1 2 **3** 4 5 6 7　WEIGHT

EXERCISE

REPS	REPS	REPS	REPS	REPS	REPS
☐	☐	☐	☐	☐	☐

1 2 3 **4** 5 6 7　WEIGHT

EXERCISE

REPS	REPS	REPS	REPS	REPS	REPS
☐	☐	☐	☐	☐	☐

1 2 3 4 **5** 6 7　WEIGHT

EXERCISE

REPS	REPS	REPS	REPS	REPS	REPS
☐	☐	☐	☐	☐	☐

1 2 3 4 5 **6** 7　WEIGHT

EXERCISE

REPS	REPS	REPS	REPS	REPS	REPS
☐	☐	☐	☐	☐	☐

1 2 3 4 5 6 **7**　WEIGHT

CARDIO

	TIME	DIST.	PACE	INT.	HR
PRE-WORKOUT					
POST-WORKOUT					

DATE: TIME:

M T W T F S S

BACK ☐ BICEPS ☐ LEGS ☐ ABS ☐
CHEST ☐ TRICEPS ☐ CALVES ☐ OTHER ☐
CARDIO ☐ FOREARMS ☐ SHOULDERS ☐

EXERCISE	REPS	REPS	REPS	REPS	REPS	REPS
1 2 3 4 5 6 7 — WEIGHT						

EXERCISE	REPS	REPS	REPS	REPS	REPS	REPS
1 **2** 3 4 5 6 7 — WEIGHT						

EXERCISE	REPS	REPS	REPS	REPS	REPS	REPS
1 2 **3** 4 5 6 7 — WEIGHT						

EXERCISE	REPS	REPS	REPS	REPS	REPS	REPS
1 2 3 **4** 5 6 7 — WEIGHT						

EXERCISE	REPS	REPS	REPS	REPS	REPS	REPS
1 2 3 4 **5** 6 7 — WEIGHT						

EXERCISE	REPS	REPS	REPS	REPS	REPS	REPS
1 2 3 4 5 **6** 7 — WEIGHT						

EXERCISE	REPS	REPS	REPS	REPS	REPS	REPS
1 2 3 4 5 6 **7** — WEIGHT						

CARDIO	TIME	DIST.	PACE	INT.	HR	
PRE-WORKOUT						
POST-WORKOUT						

DATE: | TIME:

M **T** **W** **T** **F** **S** **S**

BACK ☐ BICEPS ☐ LEGS ☐ ABS ☐
CHEST ☐ TRICEPS ☐ CALVES ☐ OTHER ☐
CARDIO ☐ FOREARMS ☐ SHOULDERS ☐

EXERCISE | REPS | REPS | REPS | REPS | REPS | REPS

1 234567 | WEIGHT

EXERCISE | REPS | REPS | REPS | REPS | REPS | REPS

1 **2** 34567 | WEIGHT

EXERCISE | REPS | REPS | REPS | REPS | REPS | REPS

12 **3** 4567 | WEIGHT

EXERCISE | REPS | REPS | REPS | REPS | REPS | REPS

123 **4** 567 | WEIGHT

EXERCISE | REPS | REPS | REPS | REPS | REPS | REPS

1234 **5** 67 | WEIGHT

EXERCISE | REPS | REPS | REPS | REPS | REPS | REPS

12345 **6** 7 | WEIGHT

EXERCISE | REPS | REPS | REPS | REPS | REPS | REPS

123456 **7** | WEIGHT

CARDIO | TIME | DIST. | PACE | INT. | HR

PRE-WORKOUT

POST-WORKOUT

DATE: | TIME:

M **T** **W** **T** **F** **S** **S**

BACK ☐ BICEPS ☐ LEGS ☐ ABS ☐
CHEST ☐ TRICEPS ☐ CALVES ☐ OTHER ☐
CARDIO ☐ FOREARMS ☐ SHOULDERS ☐

EXERCISE	REPS	REPS	REPS	REPS	REPS	REPS
1 2 3 4 5 6 7 WEIGHT						

EXERCISE	REPS	REPS	REPS	REPS	REPS	REPS
1 **2** 3 4 5 6 7 WEIGHT						

EXERCISE	REPS	REPS	REPS	REPS	REPS	REPS
1 2 **3** 4 5 6 7 WEIGHT						

EXERCISE	REPS	REPS	REPS	REPS	REPS	REPS
1 2 3 **4** 5 6 7 WEIGHT						

EXERCISE	REPS	REPS	REPS	REPS	REPS	REPS
1 2 3 4 **5** 6 7 WEIGHT						

EXERCISE	REPS	REPS	REPS	REPS	REPS	REPS
1 2 3 4 5 **6** 7 WEIGHT						

EXERCISE	REPS	REPS	REPS	REPS	REPS	REPS
1 2 3 4 5 6 **7** WEIGHT						

CARDIO	TIME	DIST.	PACE	INT.	HR	
PRE-WORKOUT						
POST-WORKOUT						

DATE:
TIME:
M T W T F S S
BACK ☐   BICEPS ☐   LEGS ☐   ABS ☐
CHEST ☐   TRICEPS ☐   CALVES ☐   OTHER ☐
CARDIO ☐   FOREARMS ☐   SHOULDERS ☐

EXERCISE
REPS   REPS   REPS   REPS   REPS   REPS
1 234567   WEIGHT

EXERCISE
REPS   REPS   REPS   REPS   REPS   REPS
1 2 34567   WEIGHT

EXERCISE
REPS   REPS   REPS   REPS   REPS   REPS
12 3 4567   WEIGHT

EXERCISE
REPS   REPS   REPS   REPS   REPS   REPS
123 4 567   WEIGHT

EXERCISE
REPS   REPS   REPS   REPS   REPS   REPS
1234 5 67   WEIGHT

EXERCISE
REPS   REPS   REPS   REPS   REPS   REPS
12345 6 7   WEIGHT

EXERCISE
REPS   REPS   REPS   REPS   REPS   REPS
123456 7   WEIGHT

CARDIO   TIME   DIST.   PACE   INT.   HR
PRE-WORKOUT
POST-WORKOUT

DATE: TIME:

M T W T F S S

BACK ☐ BICEPS ☐ LEGS ☐ ABS ☐
CHEST ☐ TRICEPS ☐ CALVES ☐ OTHER ☐
CARDIO ☐ FOREARMS ☐ SHOULDERS ☐

EXERCISE | REPS | REPS | REPS | REPS | REPS | REPS
1 234567 WEIGHT

EXERCISE | REPS | REPS | REPS | REPS | REPS | REPS
1 **2** 34567 WEIGHT

EXERCISE | REPS | REPS | REPS | REPS | REPS | REPS
12 **3** 4567 WEIGHT

EXERCISE | REPS | REPS | REPS | REPS | REPS | REPS
123 **4** 567 WEIGHT

EXERCISE | REPS | REPS | REPS | REPS | REPS | REPS
1234 **5** 67 WEIGHT

EXERCISE | REPS | REPS | REPS | REPS | REPS | REPS
12345 **6** 7 WEIGHT

EXERCISE | REPS | REPS | REPS | REPS | REPS | REPS
123456 **7** WEIGHT

CARDIO | TIME | DIST. | PACE | INT. | HR
PRE-WORKOUT
POST-WORKOUT

| DATE: | TIME: |

M T W T F S S

BACK ☐	BICEPS ☐	LEGS ☐	ABS ☐
CHEST ☐	TRICEPS ☐	CALVES ☐	OTHER ☐
CARDIO ☐	FOREARMS ☐	SHOULDERS ☐	

EXERCISE

| REPS | REPS | REPS | REPS | REPS | REPS |

1 2 3 4 5 6 7 WEIGHT

EXERCISE

| REPS | REPS | REPS | REPS | REPS | REPS |

1 **2** 3 4 5 6 7 WEIGHT

EXERCISE

| REPS | REPS | REPS | REPS | REPS | REPS |

1 2 **3** 4 5 6 7 WEIGHT

EXERCISE

| REPS | REPS | REPS | REPS | REPS | REPS |

1 2 3 **4** 5 6 7 WEIGHT

EXERCISE

| REPS | REPS | REPS | REPS | REPS | REPS |

1 2 3 4 **5** 6 7 WEIGHT

EXERCISE

| REPS | REPS | REPS | REPS | REPS | REPS |

1 2 3 4 5 **6** 7 WEIGHT

EXERCISE

| REPS | REPS | REPS | REPS | REPS | REPS |

1 2 3 4 5 6 **7** WEIGHT

CARDIO

	TIME	DIST.	PACE	INT.	HR
PRE-WORKOUT					
POST-WORKOUT					

BODY MEASUREMENTS TRACKER

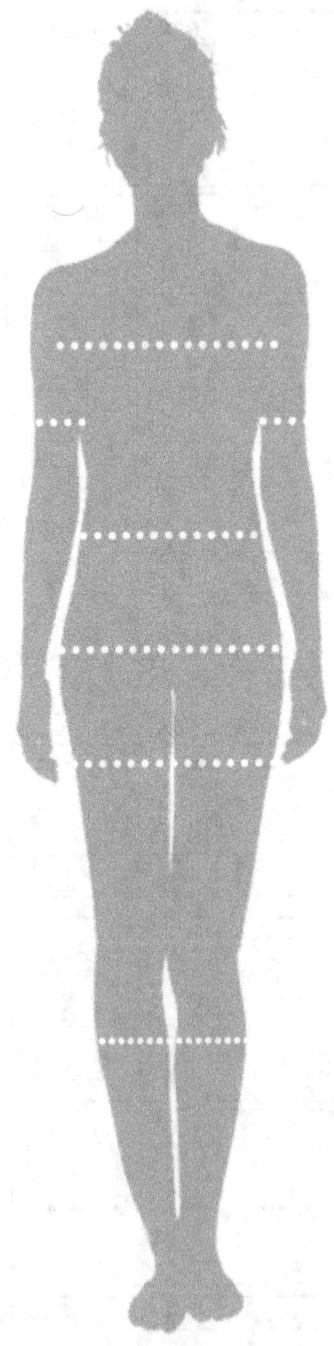

	BEFORE	AFTER
DATE		
CHEST		
LEFT ARM		
RIGHT ARM		
WAIST		
HIPS		
LEFT THIGH		
RIGHT THIGH		
LEFT CALF		
RIGHT CALF		
WEIGHT		
NOTES		

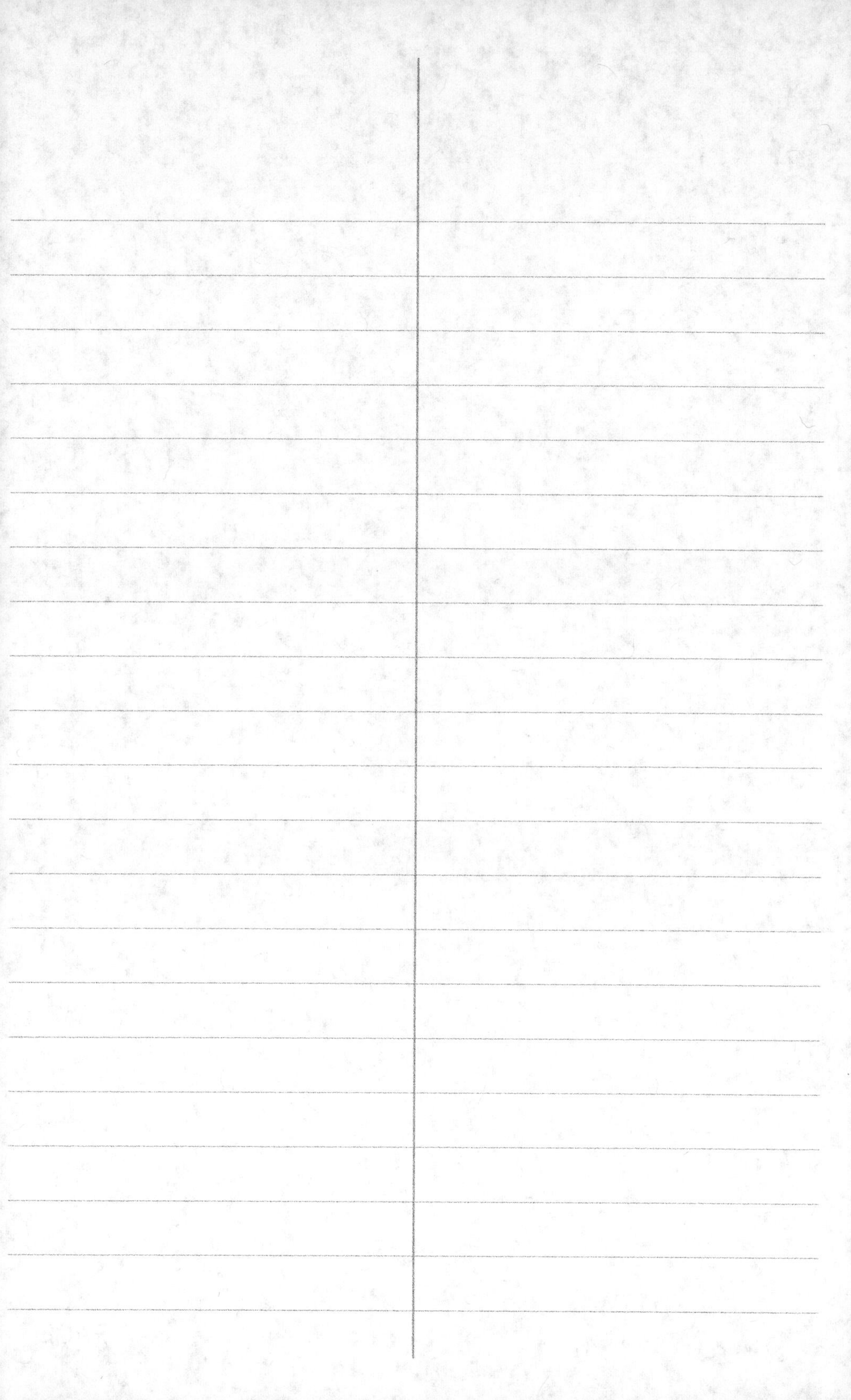

www.ingramcontent.com/pod-product-compliance
Lightning Source LLC
Chambersburg PA
CBHW061709250726

48657CB00002B/573